Living In The Magic Of Life

First Edition

By:

Yogi Vanessa

Copyright © 2019 by Vanessa Blair-Alvarez. All rights reserved.

Cover design and photo designed by Katie Thomas. All rights reserved. (on location in Ojai @Ventura Preserve)

The contents of this book may not be reproduced in any form, except for short extracts for quotation or review, without the written permission of the publisher.

The information contained within this book is strictly for spiritual educational purposes.

www.yogivanessa.com

++

Dedicated to my children, my husband, my sisters, my brother, my parents, my grandparents, ancestors, and all my friends from all over the world. And of course all my teachers, Shamans and healers from all my paths in this life. You have all had an effect on me and I am forever grateful. I send you all my infinite blessings deep into your hearts!

++

Most names and locations identified throughout this book in my stories and real situations, have been changed to respect their privacy. In the few cases where the name or identity has not been changed, I obtained their permission.

Contents

Kundalini Opening Mantra……………….....5

Foreward……………………………………..6

Introduction…………………….................22

Chapters

1. From mud pond to lotus………………31
2. Challenging Events ending in Victory…………………..................45
3. France: C'est ma vie…………………60
4. Yoga and yogic philosophy………......75
5. Magic of Learning and the Theatre………………………….....98
6. Drugs, sobriety and Reiki…………..112
7. Cannes Film Festival= Magic………127
8. Spirituality……………………………143
9. Experiences with Unexplainable Energy……………….....................159
10. Love and miracles…………………174
11. Spiritual Teacher and healer………193

Mantra

Ong Namo Guru Dev Namo

Ong = Infinite creative energy in the experience.

Namo = Same root word as in Sanskrit Namaste meaning reverent greeting.

Guru = Embodiment of the wisdom that one is seeking.

Dev = Higher, subtle or divine.

Namo = Reaffirms the humble reverence of the student.

Forward

I have been blessed since the first moment of my life, though unbeknownst to me until recently. Perhaps you are thinking I was born into a silver spoon in my mouth situation, but it was very much the opposite. I spent many years doing the inner work to heal and awaken to the higher perspective I have now in order to realize all my challenges were truly blessings. This is a huge shift from how I used to live. Being stuck in the machine of blame, depression and confusion that most of us go through in our daily lives.

It wasn't only because my alcoholic/drug addict /schizoaffective father who rejected responsibility repetitively, due to his parental circumstances, told me about the curtains in their bedroom apartment blowing apart the minute I was born, (even though the window was closed.) Nor is it because of my Jewish mother living in her own subconscious program of constant fear, as most of us do instead of constant trust, until she had enough and divorced my dad and did her inner work through discovering the church of Christian Sciences' philosophy. She attributes much of her inner success to awakening and shifting her perspectives in order to heal herself after the divorce and to raise my sister and I. Nor is it the fifteen-year old boy who molested me when I was three years old at a home daycare back in the eighties. Nor is it the elementary school that failed to see my "learning disability" and "lack of focus" issues were more profound life problems, and perhaps with an adequate public school therapist who would have recognized my issues had that been available. Lastly, it is not even the childhood debilitating asthma, that I am referring to when I say how blessed my life has been since conception.

 I recognized all these seemingly horrible life experiences as blessings and how blessed I am because my life challenges are what got me here. Each and every experience helped me grow. I begin the book with this because it is important for me YOU feel invited to begin sending signals to your own subconscious programs about how blessed even you all are thanks to the challenges presented in your lives. I wrote this book so that you can arrive to the same conclusion about your life as I have about my life; in case you have not already begun. Getting here required me to do work to arrive at a higher caliber perspective or Consciousness. Once I raised my mental caliber, through the work and experiences from Life, I was propelled to see my life with every circumstance and every life challenge as my gifts and blessings.

 I am still evolving to become even stronger, with higher caliber and with more capability of seeing pure magic blossom all around me. I plan to continue doing the joyous work because now even my perspective on work has elevated. I have studied more leaders of change and read more self-help books than I can list here, but the fastest growth for me has come from a form of yoga, called Kundalini yoga and meditation. I rejected this form of yoga after my first class at the age of seventeen, but now I see it was simply a preparation. This amazing yoga is inherently connected to my soul and as it teaches the ancient science and wisdom of yoga in every class, I could not help but to share the technology.

As I awaken through learning or remembering the ancient science of Kundalini yoga and as I continue to study all the newest science being realized by top Neuroscientists, Quantum biologists, physicists and many more healers, shamans, and medicine people of the "new age," I continue to realize that it is all correlated to the same root. Literally the question, what came first the chicken or the egg, is how I feel about the ancient science of yoga built into Kundalini yoga and meditation. Dr. Bruce Lipton Ph.D in Epigenetics and Biology clarifies so well in his book, "The Biology of Belief" how "our beliefs are creating our lives in every moment."

The technology of Kundalini yoga has been transforming my life and my beliefs about my life with every day that I continue to meditate and evolve. It has already begun to unfold outside my head and into my reality. In simply four short years of practicing and teaching Kundalini yoga and Meditation taught by Yogi Bhajan, I have weaved the puzzle pieces of information I received since childhood together to understand the really big picture that is LIFE. My beliefs have been leading me further and further down the rabbit hole to the conclusion that is, "Living In The Magic Of Life," without me being aware of it until now.

While preparing to write this book or during the writing process, I did a lot of looking back at my life to decide which stories I could share. I realized through that process that I must simply share to help others to see that their circumstances are the beginning. I feel that my story of self-awakening, my becoming more conscious and my life experiences can be relatable, helpful and potentially save one persons life. Awakening is a word that is somewhat non-tangible, right? What it is for me is a feeling of clarity through an objective observance of my own life, my own thoughts and my own stories. For those of us striving to awaken, know that you are on the right path. Every story I put into this book is what changed my life in some big way to acquire the ability to live in the magic of Life, which is an awakened state.

As I began writing this book, gathering my memories, I had to become that objective observer of my past and in doing this I experienced epiphany after epiphany. Looking back in retrospect came with ease because it was as if one experience opened me up to the next and after a while, all the magical stories from my life made me who I am today. I call it magic because some of the experiences I lived through the first time were beyond explanation in their ability to take care of me in some profound way. Remembering the stories while preparing for this book, they began re-teaching me their magic, which made last year an exceedingly magical year for me. What I have seen and the choices I have made in my life, has pushed me even further into believing in The Magic of Life. Although, there are years of stories to share, there is one potently formidable story I feel is best to share first. I chose this first example from my past because of the sheer magic that took place that afternoon. I know it will sound un-believable, but there was another person there with me to confirm it happened.

Before I share it with you, let me set an intention for you to remember to open yourself up to the possibility of change. We tend to see, hear or read things that keep us in our safe lives because our lives are comfortable and routine, but it's the change and belief in taking risks that leads us to living better lives. Being comfortable is an illusion because our lives are always changing anyway. Whether the change happens from the outside like the news, a television program that moves us to change, a friend, our society, a celebrity, or reading a book, it is all change. Therefore if you could read this next example with an open mind, in case you do not already have an open mind to see what happens.

It was a time in my life where I had been seeking my purpose and more meaning in my life. I had lived an already incredible life considering a seemingly rough beginning, as you will come to understand. The story set up begins when I had been teaching yoga privately to a group of people on the Côte d'Azur in 2002 and one of the ladies there was a model from LA. We kept in touch long afterwards and upon visiting Los Angeles, where I was from originally, I ended up hanging out with her many times. This day, she introduced me to an aura-soma therapy shop on Melrose Avenue, called Aunt Vi's Garden, which has since mysteriously closed. This is one of the many examples the Magic of Life took care of me to bring me into the realm of seeing and experiencing the Magic.

Aura-Soma therapy is a natural healing method that uses vibrational powers from crystals, color, and natural aromas combined with light. Invented by Vicki Wall, from England in the 1980's, an herbalist and gifted with "second sight" as she could see aura's. Her mind, body and Spiritual connection remained strong because her father was a deep mystic through Kabbalah and Zohar traditions and passed down his knowledge. Vicki became completely blind around the same time she created Aura-Soma readings. She explained that "unlike most therapies where the substance is chosen, Aura-Soma color bottles are chosen by the individual." The first bottle reveals who one is, the second reveals where one is coming from, the third bottle is what our mission or goals are in this life and the fourth bottle reveals what the resources are with which one may greet in life.

It was exactly the kind of place for "lost angels" like me, at that time from Los Angeles, or for people living in Los Angeles who enjoy spending time learning about the Self, discussing their horoscope, going to a psychic, receiving past life readings, doing yoga, any occult interests and any other deeper work. I had gone with her once and I chose some colors that I thought were important to me in that moment, but I was quite disappointed with my reading. Perhaps, it was because I went with someone else and there were other people in the shop, too. I could not concentrate on my intuitive voice. I could not truly feel free to choose something I may have, had I been alone.

Therefore, a year later, I went back. This time I went alone and no one was in the shop other than the guy who read the bottles. I was really trying to listen to my intuition this time and I was even asking with an intention to be shown something important. I chose 4 bottles and this time it was a lot of lavender, which I have loved since I was very young; as many of my close friends could tell you. The employee proceeded to do my reading and when he got to the full lavender bottle, he began to read what Vicki Wall had written regarding the vibrations of this color.

I was deeply enjoying what the guy was reading. With every word, I was becoming quite elevated mentally by how amazing this particular color scheme matched how I was truly feeling inside. As he began to read which herbal aroma went with this color and he opened the bottle to let me smell it, my senses were lifted even higher. He continued to talk about how the color is ruled by a certain Saint Germain, who was considered a Count back in the 17th century. He was known as an alchemist in his time and able to go forward and back in time, even though he was supposedly dead, he was seen in Paris years later. Hearing this made my mind begin to spin into asking many questions and I began to make multiple connections to thoughts I've had or books I've read like, The Alchemist, by Paulo Coelho, The Five Agreements, by Don Miguel Ruiz, A New Earth, by Eckhart Tolle, Anatomy of the Spirit, by Carolyn Myss, or my very first book into magical and mystical living, The Celestine Prophecy, by James Redfield, which I read my senior year of high school.

    Suddenly I felt an extremely strong force of energy like a tornado or strong wind pass from the wall on my left side into the store and proceed to push me towards where the store front window to the street happened to be. I was pushed so hard that I was almost lifted, without any control as if I was on a ride at Disneyland being thrown like a rag doll to the window and fell to the bench situated in front of the store's window. The guy who was giving me the reading also got pushed to the back wall of the store, which was behind the immense glass desk full of colored bottles that separated him with the register from the bottle reading counter. Immediately after hitting the window, we watched a bottle that was on a high glass shelf to my right and his left on top of the reading counter get picked up and thrown to the ground. Nothing else on that shelf moved or fell down, except for that one bottle and this whole experience there was no one was visible at all!

I began to scream out of fear as if I was watching a horror film begin in front of my eyes. I covered my ears in fear and the guy screamed, though a lot less than me, then he fell to the floor behind the counter and I couldn't see him for more than a few seconds. (On a side note, if you are the guy that worked at Aunt Vi's on Melrose Ave. can you please email or contact me immediately please because when I went back to talk to you a few months later the store had closed.) When a few seconds later the guy stood up and began to ask me if I was ok, I began to cry talk and breathe. He came out from behind the counter and he came over to me to help me up to standing because I was in total shock. He waited until I was ok and he walked back to where the bottle that had been lifted, then thrown on the ground and he announced what the bottle was titled. The name of the bottle was, "Purpose." Needless to say, I left that day in quite a state, but I bought the lavender bottle of Saint Germain nonetheless.

This experience will stay with me forever as a personal example of life's magical mystery and even as I write this story down from memory, I am moved at the visceral reality that took over my body that day. Although, I didn't understand exactly what took place, it was clear someone or something thought that I have a purpose in this life. I realize today all these years later with many hours of study about energy, yogic philosophy and quantum physics that an experience such as this isn't all that abnormal. Therefore, thanks to Saint Germain's self-imposed introduction into my life, I could no longer ignore all the invisible possibilities that lie beyond our ordinary lives. I am a being very interested in occult mystery and a seeker of answers.

Fast forward to now when another dead person came onto my radar suddenly, blessed me, and he sent me clear signs that he was contacting me to help me advance even though I did not know he was dead. His name is Dr. Wayne Dyer and he sent me three clear messages within two months time. These messages are not openly clear overt messages that any and every person would understand. They were very personal to me and only I could know and understand that he was communicating with me through these messages. It began when I was 36 weeks pregnant with my second son and about to birth in May of 2016. I had had a dream pregnancy and a miraculous surprise upon becoming pregnant when compared to my first pregnancy. I believe it was all thanks to Kundalini yoga, meditation and hypno-birthing. I became a member of Hay House emails and I received news of their annual summit. One day as my first son napped, I took the time to listen to Dr. Dyer speak during the summit. He sounded interesting and Hay House, being the great resource for self-help material that it is, was offering a movie starring Dr. Wayne Dyer called, "The Shift." A few days before my son began his arrival, I watched "The Shift."

    What a lovely film to watch just before I would birth this miracle boy into my life. The film infused me with high frequency vibes and the arrival of my second son was a successful home birth and truly a dream birthing experience. The miracles and the magic that I will discuss, share and basically prove in the following chapters, is available for all humans upon their choosing. How do I know I can prove this? I have done it for myself as a radical skeptic on more than one occasion. In fact a month after the birth of my son, I decided to ask Dr. Dyer to show himself to me in a way that I would know it was him.

I had already begun writing some chapters of my book at that time, but I was very stuck about how to share and ask for help. A day after my request, I received an email from Hay House saying that I qualified for a free e-book. All I had to do was choose from a list of authors and to my happy surprise one of the titles was by Dr. Dyer. It was his book, "Wishes Fulfilled" that I chose. This would prove to be his second time contacting me to help me in advance. "Wishes Fulfilled," had become another pivotal moment in my life that propelled me into confidence, belief, and stunned awe that the Magic of Life was not only working for me but also lifting me towards my new self.

The third contact was inside the book, "Wishes Fulfilled" which I read in a week, even with a newborn baby. I couldn't nap with the baby, nor with my first son because I only wanted to read. In Dr. Dyer's book, he deeply discusses Saint Germain's life and I was thinking the whole time, "okay Dr. Dyer, okay Saint Germain, I get it and thank you." I had not thought about Saint Germain in over twelve years. He was telling me more about Saint Germain's life as a way of contacting me. He conveyed his message to me to relax into our connection because he would be available to help me from then on and it was not a coincidence. That was Dr. Dyer's way of clarifying to me his message that he was available to help me further my book and that he wanted this book to succeed. His way of confirming yet again that Living in the Magic of Life is always possible.

After reading "Wishes Fulfilled" for the first time, I went and looked up more information about Dr. Dyer and his life. I didn't know how he passed on or why I would never have the chance to meet him in person. After reading about him, I went back to re-read, "Wishes

Fulfilled" only to discover the answer to my disappointment of never being able to meet him in person. This was his final way of solidifying our connection because he was literally explaining to me how he needed to be in another realm in order to reach me as I was looking to believe in the Magic.

In the first chapter of his book, he writes about being more than an ordinary person to obtain all that we want to manifest in our lives. We must be or realize we are extraordinary. He writes, "…extraordinary consciousness is associated with your soul, that invisible, boundaryless energy that looks out from behind your eyeballs and has very different interests than your ordinary self does.

The ideal of your soul, the thing that it yearns for, is not more knowledge. It is not interested in comparison, nor winning, nor light, nor ownership, nor even happiness. The ideal of your soul is space, expansion, and immensity, and the one thing it needs more than anything else is to be free to expand, to reach out and to embrace the infinite. Why? Because your soul is infinity itself. It has no restrictions or limitations—it resists being fenced in— and when you attempt to contain it with rules and obligations, it is miserable."

After re-reading this portion, I received his answer. He said that it was because his soul was without restriction in this form and he can help more people; in the same way he was helping me. It was so clear that he is supporting me in my life, but what he proved to me was that this type of relationship is possible. He confirmed what had happened to me more than ten years prior in that aura-soma shop on Melrose Ave. that invisible beings are available to help us on this plane and what could be more magical than that? It reminds me of the Asian cultures tradition of leaving food, flowers, and incense for the spirits passed on. They believe that, why can't we?

I now realize without a shadow of a doubt that every seeming challenge in my life was to question me into changing my perception. These unbelievable things that happened to me, allowed me to question my beliefs. Through questioning everything, I grew and I learned about my mind and the illusion of societies' reality. When I remain in the magic and the joy of Life, I am not knocked or pushed to the ground by the challenges. I now see how the magic works and I can see my whole life as a blessing. I can even understand my parents based on what their parents taught them or even understand how to forgive a child molester.

Forgiveness is part of healing our Self and is also a concept to learn deep in our being as an experience, so that we are able to live in the magic of life. Getting to forgiveness took 20 years, but it has chiseled me into the human I am today living a life so magical and so amazing. I finally believe the story my biological dad told me about the moment I was born. I am now able to live blissfully through days filled with magic and not worry about the seeming troubles of the moment with my kids, or husband, or the president. It is always our choice whether we choose to continue believing our subconscious story or continue to blame our parents, friends and society for the way we think. My whole life was always pushing me forward into a new paradigm of understanding where magic is the way to see life.

In this book, I want to explain how the sum total of my life experiences brought me to the magic and show you that it is absolutely possible for you. No matter where you are at in your life, it can begin today. All the work you've already done can be capitalized upon to fulfill yourself and re-calibrate your thinking with a kind of re-birth experience that you might be able to say your life, with all the pain, struggle, fear and worry is also a blessing. Reading this book from start to finish may be exactly your Magical life beginning to take hold of you to lead you to your highest Self.

    A final example I will share with you as proof that I have traversed many challenges, but have chosen to see them as ways to strengthen myself and believe that what ever does not kill me makes me stronger was when I faced my own death for the first time at age twelve. One of the scariest nights of my childhood came in the form of an asthma attack. I was attending Jane Fonda's performing arts camp called, "Laurel Springs" above Santa Barbara, where we had opportunities to do theatre, dance, photography, painting, swimming, feed farm animals and be around other kids doing the same thing. I loved it there and I had a huge crush on her son, Troy, too. One night we were forced to camp outside our cabins under the stars and hike to our camping spot after the sun went down. Soon after leaving our bunks, I realized that I had forgotten my inhaler. For anyone with asthma, you know that having an inhaler with you at all times, is an absolute must.

    Before allowing my anxiety to take over, as it was too late already because my attack was already too strong, I began to internally ask for help. I made a choice to simply cure myself. I became a true self-healer because of something inside that led me to teach myself to breathe in a specific way through the anxiety of possible death. I was blessed because hearing my intuition speak to me and coach me on how to breathe deeply, even though my lungs could not take in any air, was enough for me do the work. In my mind, I had to do that or die. Focusing on the stars and breathing very slowly through the mucous or anxiety or whatever asthma is, I was able to calm down and stop my wheezing enough to fall asleep in peace. That was the first time in my whole life that I didn't have to go to the hospital with an attack that bad.

For anyone who's never experienced an asthma attack, it feels much like ones' chest is going to implode and no air will pass. Then, an anxiety takes over all mental energy because the fear begins to take over. Finally, you realize you cannot inhale but only gasp for air unless you get a puff from an inhaler to clear the lungs from their seeming blockages. Not having my prized inhaler that night was meant to be. I faced a serious challenge that would, in retrospect, help me realize all these years later that I am a natural born healer and we all can be!

Wow, simply the re-description of this experience brings me back into that state of anxiety because my muscles, body and cells remember so well. I must say that I agree with Dr. Bruce Lipton Ph.D about how our cells remember everything through the feelings we feel in our body. He is an amazing Biologist that I studied with at Quantum University online based on his book, "The Biology of Belief." Dr Bruce Lipton also gives talks all around the world based on his findings about Biology, cells, DNA and epigenetics. His research and findings about how our minds are much more powerful than we previously understood is now the most current science along with quantum physics.

Not to get over scientific on you, but our emotions are how the brain builds neuro pathways from synapses inside that brain which release a chemical into our blood stream after one neuron fires to the next based on our memory and beliefs. This is according to a neurologist Dr. Joe Dispenza, who I have also studied ever since seeing a film called, "What the Bleep Do We Know" back in 2004. He introduced the most fascinating way of understanding our brain, mind and body in how it correlates to how we create our current realities. Dr. Dispenza introduced me to the idea that we can talk to our psyche and our electromagnetic field to influence how our reality plays out as a co-creation all those years ago in 2004. That movie was one of my favorites of all time because it was the first eye-opening example of something I had known deep inside of me at my core. Little did I know back then, that eleven years later, I would experience the reality of this practice when I became a Kundalini yoga and meditation teacher and student.

Yogi Bhajan, the Kundalini yoga master that brought this ancient form of yogic technology to the West, knew all of this forty years before the movie even came out. He experienced the truth of this as early as six years old and knew he had to share this truth with the West. What he brought for us to practice concurs with and even goes beyond what I learned from Dr. Joe Dispenza Ph.D and Dr. Bruce Lipton Ph.D because Yogi Bhajan does not separate one science from another. Kundalini yoga is what scientists, quantum physicists, and quantum bioenergeneticists have only recently begun to describe and observe in their tests as truth. It occurred to me that after all my years of seeking help, researching, studying from various self-help authors, doctors, healers, shaman, etc, I had finally found a real way to heal myself at the deepest level. It is through using Kundalini yoga and meditation mixed with the science of eating sattvic foods and keeping up with my practice that I could achieve living in the Magic of Life daily. This is a life long process of constant inner awareness mixed with outer faith and listening to my intuition to continue to heal all my past lives and unconscious beliefs that I still have in my mind.

I became a Power yoga teacher in 2002 because the physical practice got me excited. There is something to the doing of yogic asanas in any form of yoga that initiates a true self-awareness and outer world awakening. I grew up dancing and competing in dancing until the age of 15 when I totally gave up my passion of dancing. I had formed an idea of my physical self in dance classes that was based on the consciousness of the times. In dance, we are taught to be self aware of our outer body and how it looks in a mirror, but that always kept me in a vicious cycle of never feeling confident. When I stopped dancing, I was able to begin to climb my mental ladder of punishment and reward to discover a truer truth about myself little by little.

When I tried yoga for the first time at 17, I quickly understood how the asanas created a way to use the physical body to go beyond our old thoughts and breathe. My Power yoga teacher explained and taught methods in every class on how to breath through any and all challenges that he suggested with postures. It was in taking in the prana, "life force," which helped me to truly bridge my outside physical body to the inside of my body. The yoga began healing me right from the beginning at seventeen on many levels, but it was a subtle process. I had been well programmed by the collective society, because even when I tried Kundalini at seventeen and again at twenty, it was too "weird" for my young age, until the program of society literally stopped working for me.

Through my personal yogic journey beginning with Power yoga as a student to teaching it and then discovering Kundalini yoga, which always includes meditation, I was constantly awakening to the magic, no matter how long it took to get me there. It took twenty years of studying all the myriad of philosophies and self-help methods and twenty years of trying out all those methods to begin to receive the right information. The information constantly being given by my intuition, but that I was taught to ignore. Therefore, it was truly when I began teaching Kundalini yoga and meditation that all the answers I had always been asking began to flow into my life like a faucet. Kundalini yoga wasn't like the little tastes that I had been given over the years, but a full on constant auto renewal of awareness, opportunity and awakening. My life is now in the "zone" of ever-evolving magic and flow; and I am sure it is thanks to Kundalini yoga and meditation

I have chosen a salt and pepper mixture of philosophies to explain my discovery of living in the magic of life because I believe there is more than one method for one to evolve. Religion, siblings, children, deaths, parents, college, discussions with friends, meeting people with stories, yoga classes, music, books, Ted talks and more are some of the different nuggets of wisdom to collect on all of our journey's to our highest path.

I have finally fulfilled my life long desire to know my truth and realize my purpose, which helped me begin to see all my blessings over the last 39 years. All these years later, I understand how breathing through an asthma attack wasn't the first big challenge/ blessing in my life, but it was a continuum of my ever unfolding journey towards self-realization. This new level of irrevocable self-awakening allows life to feel extraordinary and magical every single day. This is the beginning towards "Living In The Magic Of Life" and this is my "rags to riches" story and my way to serve humanity.

Introduction

To experience the magic of life, as I am describing in this book, one must simply be ALIVE. Once that is established and obvious, I believe, we are all capable to live everyday in the "magic of life." In fact, we are supposed to live with an invisible and magical hand lifting us towards the next activity, meeting, and experience to help our souls advance. The magic, I am referring to, is not smoke and mirrors or woo-woo like in certain definitions. I like two definitions that I will repeat here from my Iphone dictionary: "2. The art of producing a desired effect or result through the use of incantation or various other techniques that, presumably assure human control of supernatural agencies or the forces of nature. 6. Any extraordinary or mystical influence, charm, power, etc." These two definitions of magic simply touch upon the kind of magical life I know is possible for everyone. Why do I believe it is possible for all humans, because one, I am living it right now and because two, one cannot understand magical living without experiencing it. What I call magical living defies our societal reality or collective consciousness, (or "Maya" as we call it in yogic philosophy.)

In Maya, or some call it the matrix, the field, life, or reality, not everyone will allow themselves to believe in a life full of magic because it does not fit the prescribed path that we are taught from our parents, teachers, society or the media. Maya currently says, grow up, get rich by doing well in school or other methods, getting into a good college, getting a good job that makes you rich or even become media famous, marry someone beautiful, have beautiful kids, a beautiful dog, a beautiful cat, put beautiful photos up on social media to prove you've succeeded in the societal game and when it's time to die, utilize all the medical/ pharmaceutical care available, but be as quiet and private as you can. This is a glitch in our matrix. This description of life is not what my book is about because I believe that description is not only fraudulent, but the opposite to living in the feeling of a magical life.

For most of you, you already know what I am talking about, but for many of you it might be time to let go of this archetype or life mold, even if you have successfully accomplished it. If you cannot do that, then simply take the rest of this book as my perspective or my story and then create your opinion. I am asking you now and for the remainder of this book to go behind Maya and the curtain of society into the Matrix. I ask you to do this for the benefit of finding your own magical life.

All magic is uniquely personal to the individual. I cannot begin to define how your life will look, living in YOUR magical life because only you can do that once you've discovered being in the magical zone. Although, I can express how it may feel. It will feel as if your most inner secret/ purpose in life is lifting you up and flying you around like being on a magic carpet carrying you from new experience to new experience. You will feel a deep subtle confidence carrying you and surrounding you, like an aura, every day.

When something comes up that is challenging, no matter what it is, an inner confidence activates and like a tennis match you know you will win; the challenge will invigorate you to move beyond where you are standing. The confidence instills itself in all your cells through the challenges because you know that learning, growing and becoming stronger into your purpose is the only outcome. Every moment feels as if it were your personal synchronistic moment helping you to become more authentically you living with instant manifestations popping into existence along the way. I am reminded of horoscopes as an example of remaining confident through the challenges. Whenever someone announces that Saturn is visiting, people always get nervous because it means challenges may arise, but Saturn is present to teach important life lessons in a new way. It's like if someone gave you a kingdom and told you to be the king or queen, could you rise to the challenge and win or simply reject it because it sounds too hard or crazy?

    Another way to experience living in the magic of life is to begin a program dedicated to self-help and self-awareness, which might question all or some of your current beliefs. A wonderful fast track program is Kundalini yoga and meditation, which you will see and perhaps begin to do in this book. I lead you to Kundalini yoga because when I re-discovered it presented to me for the fourth time, I felt, it was the defining moment of my life asking me to live inside a solid trust tunnel made of this magic. I have never wanted to say yes to anything more in my life. Feeling our magical life unfolding around us in every moment is the realest life for humans on this planet. I will share an easy meditation with you now that if done for 40 days is said to make the impossible possible. Maybe try it after this chapter or follow it now if you are feeling called to move into meditation and then come back for the rest of the chapter.

Meditation:
<u>Gan Puttee Kriya</u>
"To make the impossible possible"

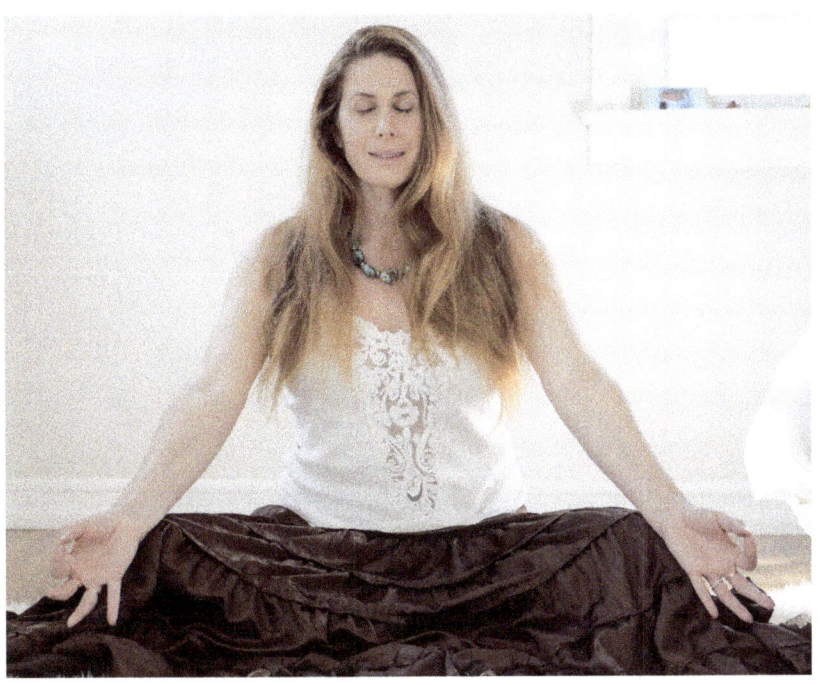

Sa- thumb to pointer finger (Jupiter)	Ta- thumb to middle finger (Saturn)
Na- thumb to ring finger (Sun)	Ma- thumb to pinkie finger (Mercury)
Ra- thumb to Jupiter finger	Ma- thumb to Saturn finger
Da- thumb to Sun finger	Sa- thumb to Mercury finger
Sa- thumb to Jupiter finger	Say- thumb to Saturn finger
So- thumb to Sun finger	Hung- thumb to Mercury finger

Begin with 11 minutes of reciting these words while touching the fingertips together with every chant of each word. Begin sitting down in easy pose like a yogi with spine straight. To finish: inhale and hold for up to 30 seconds while you move the rest of your body vigorously, then exhale. Do it two more times just as this first time.

"This redeems all the negativity of your past and present. It will take away all negative karma of your past, smooth out your daily problems and create a positive tomorrow."

I also believe that reading self-help books is an essential technique for hearing new philosophies or quite literally, methods towards achieving and living an authentically magical life. Most individuals will naturally gravitate towards an aspect of self-help or author that is perfect for them in that moment of evolution and this is where the self-help magic begins; it's much like the law of attraction. Something I'm sure most of you have already heard of in your lives. You will attract or be attracted to the type of self-help concept based on what area you need most help in at that time. This is the first step towards living in your magic because only you know what area is the most pertinent for you in your evolution.

The information to help oneself change a perspective depends on that individual, as we are all dealing with different issues at different moments thanks the this matrix that holds us all together in one world. Essentially self-help books explain a new concept that aids you to get on a new path to think and live differently, or at least introduce new ideas to consider. This is a necessity for all of us to find our "magic." We always need new ideas and concepts to challenge our belief system about reality, otherwise how can we grow?

How many of you have heard of a book, but it took months to actually get it and read it? On the contrary, how many of you were dealing with a life problem and a friend handed you a book you read that same day? Coming to understand that it was exactly what you needed to change your life perspective in that moment of your life. That's the magic of the law of attraction, but it's only one layer to living in the magic of life. For me, self-help books were on my ladder towards renewing my life since middle school. Learning many methods of self-help to achieve a clear minded, healthy and higher vibrational way of thinking has brought me to be the person I am today, which is the person I have waited for since I was born.

  To be clear, everything I have experienced in my short life has led me to write this book. I feel it is important to express, that half of my purpose is to share my life with humanity because we are one. Therefore, if one of us has discovered something important that could impact all of humanity in a great way, than it must be shared. That is my personal belief to help humans awaken to their own magic. Inside I am constantly opening to what I have to do to achieve my purpose and how to think about it along the way. I am lucky, but I searched for a long time.

  For you all who read this, it may not begin as an obvious shift at first, but if you try the meditations and perhaps begin to modify your perspective, a feeling or sense of your purpose will arise for you, as well. That is when challenges will begin to no longer feel a need to be categorized as good, bad, challenging, scary, or unnecessary in your subconscious or conscious mind. Life then becomes so magical that you can start to see yourself as the artist of your own life with all the colors and emotions representing old categories of self judgement that get alchemized. Becoming hyper aware of who you are inside will be the beginning step.

I organized 11 major life situations that I feel portray, such as my story from the foreward, my beliefs and my achievements on how life can be magical if you choose to believe. I will describe them in the following chapters to explain how I got to this perspective on magic being real and not just a myth or concept. I honestly believe life is magical for everyone in every moment because I can see it, even when others cannot. Breaking life up into its moments makes being objective easier for us all and we can start to realize it is those moments that can be considered as magical. One moment leads to the next, then to the next and so on until, all day long magic is transpiring. That is why the present moment is a gift!

It was these 11 life experiential concepts that created what I had been seeking and learning all my life to be profoundly magical upon my awakening to the truth of Life. I didn't walk on water or levitate, yet, but the power I gained from these special experiences turned the light on for me; first dimly and now it is brighter than the sun. Allow me to present an idea regarding the new paradigm arriving on our planet so that it can emerge for everyone in a powerful way. Magic is the energy that has always been kept secret, but with the current paradigm shifting from patriarchal to matriarchal, from Piscean to Aquarian, we are all being asked to upgrade in every way.

You might think, perhaps she is a presumptuous person to say she lived through something comparable to walking on water or even magic. Who am I to judge something I've seen, heard, experienced and call it magical? Well, "I am that I am," as Dr. Wayne Dyer Ph.D says in his book, "Wishes Fulfilled" and as Moses says in the Torah. When he asked the burning bush how to call God, God responded, "I am that I am." We are all what we say and think we are, but most of us are not aware of it. When I realized that I am the judge of my own life, I began to choose in every moment whether I am conscious or running on a subconscious program that I developed during childhood. This is confirmed in ancient science and new psychology as well; we all record our lives from age zero to six. Then we live with the programs from that age.

On the cusp of the new paradigm called the Age of Aquarius, we are still reacting like we are in the old paradigm where we were all socialized and taught to have judgments of others in our society from an outside perspective rather than to accept others or look inside our Self first. Looking inside our self is a muscle to be developed and the byproduct is compassion. Once we can live in compassion for ourselves, we can act with compassion towards humans. This new paradigm is subtly inviting us to transform our old ways into something more aware.

The path towards more self-awareness is infused into the information age. It exists to create pressure and stimulation through social media, the news, all marketing constantly presented to us via commercials, billboards, facebook/ instagram ads, etc. and it all creates a feeling of stress and overwhelm to the point that we cannot clearly see true importance in our lives. Once this pressure is so strong that we all feel bombarded in similar ways, perhaps we will learn how to rebel by creating silence. In the silence we can better listen to our inner wisdom and that will allow overall compassion to bloom. Compassion is another level towards Living in the Magic of Life.

Perhaps, if our society started teaching us at conception, birth, or in pre-school to be open to the idea that there is an infinite amount of experiences possible, we might begin to accept the unexplainable as normal; instead of calling it magic. We will all learn during this new paradigm of the myriad possibilities within energy, science, the mind, our beliefs and everything unseen and start to use magic as an everyday vernacular. On that tangent, if our society taught us how to feel the energy within ourselves from our inside life force (prana) or from all the energy outside of our bodies, (electromagnetic field) then perhaps our society would understand and we could shift the paradigm faster. Perhaps we are not there yet, for we are in the cusp period, but perhaps I'm writing this to say that we're closer than I think…? One thing is sure we are all in this together.

Chapter 1

From mud pond to lotus

"There is the mud, and there is the lotus that grows out of the mud. We need the mud in order to make the lotus."
      Thich Nhat Hanh

Born in Santa Monica on Seventh Street in my parents' bedroom certainly set me up well as a Southern California angel. Los Angeles was where I picked to incarnate in 1977. I was an innocent little baby with a big soul purpose. I was born with no idea of my dad's mental issues and my soul chose him as my birth father anyway. (Yogi's believe along with many other Eastern philosophies that our soul chooses our parents, siblings, our lives and our circumstances to transform us and to pay off our karma for our growth all before birth.) By the time I was four, we had already moved from my birth apartment in Santa Monica to a house on Walnut Street in Venice and again to an apartment in Santa Monica. As soon as I was able to be somewhat independent, around age three, I began to travel around my neighborhood. I had an intense inner desire to know my surroundings and enough confidence to get out of the house on my own. One funny story that my mother will tell people is that when I was three years old, I would push a chair up to the door of our apartment, climb up onto it and unlock the door by myself. She would find me outside somewhere playing or at a neighbor's house. Can we talk about limit testing!

I got to know all the people in the neighborhood by name around where we lived. I was so curious to discover and to introduce myself to meet everyone. I remember some neighbors from my street and knowing the liquor store owner two streets up. I suppose all this was just to get outside and see the world. It was an inner drive in me to do things that I probably should not have been doing at three. I felt an enormous push or inner mission to be out discovering and socializing.

It's probably a miracle that I never got hurt or kidnapped, but nonetheless my stubborn nature was teaching me to trust an inner sense of personal intuition.

Now as I think back in retrospect, I realize after years of therapy, years of natural medicine, years of self-help, self-analysis and studying psychology that, I was out in the world watching how other families and people functioned. As if I was studying people to develop my energetic tool kit of discernment, then I measured and gauged from what I was seeing in my own family life. It was simply another example of the Magic of Life taking care of me by using my capacities to get away from the household tension in my home. By the time I was eight my parents had been divorced for four years and I remember being indifferent to their divorce. It was probably because I was so young and couldn't emotionally process all that my life was throwing at me, but on some inner level I knew it was meant to be. One memory I will never forget happened before school, when I was in elementary school. Most memories are categorized by being extraordinarily great, traumatic, or too shocking the mind puts it deep into the dark psyche. This memory was more traumatic and almost too shocking because it is still painful on an emotional level for me. In my little girl mind, I was in danger and things were not kosher for me on a foundational comfort. That morning, my dad was upset and yelling at my mom, which was already quite abusive. Then he picked up the breakfast I had been eating on top of one of those big plastic crates and threw it at me. I was so scared and did not understand, but more importantly I didn't feel safe.

I was scarred by that morning and by my home life in general. It must have been clear to me that my home life was abusive to me developing a healthy psyche for a young girl in this world. I deducted that I could not rely on adults to do, say, and create the harmonious environments I was wishing for deep within. I was also calculating how to be safe after the memory and experience of being molested at home pre-school when I was three by the woman's son. Another traumatic experience that I still to this day have no recollection how it happened, but deep within me I have worked on transmuting the trauma many times.

    My body reacted to all the uncertainty and abuse by creating terrible asthma. Why is this pertinent for me to share? Mostly because as Dr. Bruce Lipton Ph.D. alludes to in his book, "The Biology of Belief," my young mind created this biological symptom, asthma, as a signal that I could not think straight. I literally did not believe my life was safe. The asthma was so bad that I had to repeat kindergarten after half way through my first year around I was going to the hospital or asthma doctor every other day. Concentrating on learning from a book was not a priority for me at that time when my childhood life was overwhelmingly complicated. Frankly, I was probably in survivor mode thinking I could only stay with my mother or else I would not be safe. At that age, my mind was not online yet and kids aren't able to make clear choices that would impact daily routine in a real way. They were sort of stuck with the choices of their parents and most kids handle it, but I was not like most kids. I had life situations other than school constantly distracting me and I ended up learning to cope by having asthma attacks when I felt too overwhelmed.

    As I started to grow up and entered Franklin Elementary, I learned to distract my fear and grief by being trying to be social. I made friends, but it was a struggle. My parents were divorced and all of my friends had parents still together. Most of my friends lived in huge houses and we lived in an apartment. All I was confronted with made me rise to the occasion or feel defeated and depressed. I had peers who traveled around the world and came back telling me their stories. I found a way into relating to their stories by using my imagination and because of my deep inner desire of discovering new places. I would listen to their stories and inside I would imagine myself doing what they described and more. International travel was totally a foreign experience to me at eight years young. Some kids would come to school with stories about seeing the pyramids in Egypt, the Eiffel Tower in France or even a friend who was from Japan and brought us rice candy covered in edible paper. I was too young to realize, but I began to believe I would have those same experiences.

    My first time on a plane that I remember, was to Texas to visit my grandparents. I wasn't super excited to visit my grandparents, but I was excited to be going to a new place to discover. I remember this particular flight because I was alone with my younger sister and she was having trouble with her ears and the air pressure. The flight attendant gave me two plastic cups with wet warm paper towels in bottom of each and told me to hold them tightly over her ears. It was the experience of caring for her in that plane that etches that experience into my memory. Although caring for my sister was something I was used to, being the oldest, I had already decided at a young age it was my job to care for her, as I thought my mother could not. I loved that airplane experience because it made me confident in my ability to be independent.

Being in a plane above the clouds quickly became one of my most magical places in the world. I always look out the windows and feel closer to something divine while being amongst the clouds, close to the galaxy and in the open blue skies. From realizing that being in a plane gave me that feeling of beginners mind where the impossible becomes a possibility, I knew I was destined to do a lot more of that in my life without worrying about the timing. That experience of taking care of my sister successfully gave me a place of confidence to enjoy and re-imagine over and over in my mind. Even though my outward life felt tragic, somehow the magic of life began to lift me up. I developed an unwavering optimism despite all the darkness.

What I didn't know at my young age was that my mother was going through her own magical self-healing time. She was getting out of a bad divorce with the responsibility of two young daughters and living far from her own family. It was her introduction to Christian Science that would eventually save her and reverberate into saving my sister and me. She had to begin to change her own beliefs about life, religion, community, family and perhaps the fact that she was in charge of uplifting herself. Somehow her struggle permeated my psyche on a very subtle level and helped me improve my perspective about life. This is when the Magic truly began to support me in a real way.

My mom dated a few guys after her divorce that I remember and each one brought something better to our lives. Meeting people makes an impression that can be indelible in the mind of a child. My sister and I were constantly learning about life through our parents' struggles and no matter how unsafe or scared we felt, we were being shaped by the world around us. At eight and a half years old, I had lived through many challenges in my short life, but my mom made her final decision, which would affect our lives forever forward.

I remember meeting Philippe for the first time; the man who would ultimately become my Step Father. At that age, I was a candy conaisseuse, thanks to one of my neighbor friends whose father was the inventor of gummy worms. The flavor of those gummy worms formed my taste buds towards gummy candy and candy in general. Tastes have a way of creating memories in our mind and act as place markers as an almost visceral reaction during that time of our lives. This friend of mine, Danielle, who I no longer have contact with will forever remain a strong memory from the time I lived on Berkeley street. I was either at her house playing or else I was at King's liquor buying "abba-zabbas" or "whatchamacallits." My Step Father made the genius decision to bring my sister and I a surprise that first time we met him that he hid in the fridge. He told us we had to look for it. When we finally found it, it was called a "look" bar and it was a kind of candy I had never seen. I loved him from that first impression, knowing he had star quality in my eyes.

As life would attract to me, thanks to my burgeoning magical belief system and imagination, it turned out Philippe, the guy with the funny name like the horse from "Beauty and the Beast," was Belgian. His family lived in France, but he was born in Zaire, Africa because his great grand father owned a coffee and tea plantation where his father made coffee and tea. Life had given me more than just a vacation trip to another country to experience, it gifted me an entire culture. Magic gave me a portal and a lifestyle to deeply experience for my life and to form my own destiny.

I consider Philippe my true father even though I met him at the age of eight and three quarters. My biological dad and I made many memories because he had visitation whenever he was available, but he was not the one who was there day in and day out, that was Philippe. My biological father took my sister and I to many movies, taught us surfing and to his apartment where he set up an easel to paint while he played guitar and sang and he bought us mice to play with. They are good memories etched in my mind, but because he did not live with us, nor did he make a choice to become mentally healthy, it became clear to me much later on in my life that the little we did receive from him was a blessing because it was his best.

Philippe began to live with us and as far as I was concerned, he was already my father simply by his presence in our apartment. Not long after he was living with us, I made a decision to commit to learning how to communicate in French because of Philippe. Thanks to Philippe, I was interested in his history and it was my green light to learn about the world. It was fascinating to discover how the Belgians were kicked out of Zaire, Africa by President Moboutu. I did a report on Zaire in Seventh grade and I received the highest grade of my entire scholastic career. Upon learning more about Philippe as the years continued, I learned about his father and mother, André and Delmarmol. After a while in Zaire, André was forced to choose from only two options, after being forced to leave, either go back to Belgium or go to the south of France where Philippe's grandfather had over 150 acres of land. There was an old house and old barn buildings, fruit trees, olive trees and some grapes on that land.

André chose the South of France and turned that piece of land into an award-winning vineyard in less than 50 years. He poured his whole life into the land, the grapes, the weather, the dirt, the animals and the outcome of a good bottle of wine. I was able to develop a great taste for good wine and not good wine thanks to André's amazing red wine, Chevalier. He died during the writing of this book, but he was and will always be a huge part of the best magic from my life. It's so rare to have the opportunity to know a person of his caliber, moreover work along side a human so connected to the earth.

André was my step-grandfather, but we had such an interesting rich relationship. He taught me true integrity, self-respect, diplomacy, strength, assertiveness and self-protection. He used to tease me to the point of tears, but as the years went on and I got to know him better, I realized exactly how he felt about me. He knew how strong-minded I was and he wanted to test me to become stronger out of a deep love for my inner convictions. He was molding me into a better, stronger, more capable human. He was very generous to me and he was a living example, as opposed to something we learn in school or a book and then try to understand with experience. I learned from him first hand for over twenty years, but even more towards the end of his life. I worked for him at the Vineyard for a few years and we became very close. He was a man of principal and dignity. He would tell me, "the nouveau rich people have no idea about life."

André's family was Belgian royalty from many generations and lifetimes before. His family crest derived from the kings' horsemen and having that heritage shaped him in certain ways. Even with that as his foundation, he still made mistakes to learn from in his life. Towards the end of his life, I began to see that in his own way, he understood his mistakes and felt the deep consequences of his acts, despite never changing the karma. As most people from older generations do, he stayed true to a certain level of integrity and pride even without asking for forgiveness or apologizing. Being able to stand near a man of that caliber and watching how life mistakes shape a person and a family has taught me so much about how to have immense gratitude for my life and about the importance of forgiveness. André's life could teach much of humanity a thing or two about having power while being a humble human, just as his life was an example for me. I miss him deeply.

 Life really set me up well as it turned out with this funny guy named, Philippe. As a magical life would have it, Philippe also had two kids. One of which was his oldest daughter who was "that girl in my after school day care who liked lentil soup." I think I played next to her a few times but we were not friends. I don't remember the exact day Philippe brought his kids over to meet us, but since that day, we have been family good, bad, and all.

 I do remember the day Philippe moved into our apartment "for good." The four kids went and played at the park just across the street from his "bachelor pad." We had no idea what was happening, but we didn't care because there were swings and slides. Kids are very resilient and we just accepted everything happening to us. From then on, we grew up building forts with our two couches' pillows and sheets, sliding down the stairs of our three-story apartment on pillows, and creating new "Cirque Du Soleil" choreography every weekend. My clothes got passed down to my stepsister and she passed them back down to the next sister. My stepbrother played Barbie's with us, dressed up to dance with us during our "Cirque Du Soleil" shows and even if he was un-happy he was in our gang. We also went through sibling challenges as most siblings do, but I am so grateful that we are still family.

Life was just beginning to prepare me in a way that I knew deep down it could after such a rough beginning, but never believed it would. After a few years, Philippe and my mom got married and all us kids were in the wedding. Around that time, I was twelve and made a decision that he was my real dad without ever telling him, but it was an unconscious decision. I realize now it was a decision, which displays my inner personality about self-protection, self-preservation and deep openness toward others. He made an impression on me to a point that I wanted to be connected to someone and feel I had a father.

As a complete 180° turn around and fast-forward to the writing of this book, in total shock to me, my biological father also died during the writing and editing of this book. I hadn't spoken to or seen him since November 2015. The decision that I made so long ago about Philippe was questioned when my biological father died earlier this year. I realized that the bond one maintains in the body with a blood parent is truly unconditional. We did have a unique father daughter relationship with fun and loving memories, but after we both reached a certain age (and the many disappointments, betrayals, and my own self protection,) I couldn't make excuses for him anymore. I had to distance myself from him because it put me in too much pain and sadness whenever I did see him, but I did and will always love him.

He was mentally un-stable and even though in my early years I thought going to movies, the arcade and getting to listen to him play his electric bumble bee painted guitar while my sister and I painted, was awesome, he was a life long depressive. When someone is so broken by their life situation, they unconsciously decide between two options, fix one self and heal or stay broken. As most of us who are hurt or stuck in our pain, we sometimes have a victim mindset. He had been alcohol sober since my younger full blood sister was born, about thirty-five years, but even sobriety did not heal him.

My sister and I grew up going to AA, al-anon meetings and hearing him repeat his prayers everyday, but he failed to believe that his own happiness was the goal. However, the twelve steps were not enough for my dad to change his core beliefs. The eleventh step, which is meditation, fails to truly teach humans how to meditate for the brain, grey matter, and synapses that facilitate repetitive behavior patterns. I watched a broken human choose to stay broken and die broken. His example has shaped me and given me the motivation to find alternative methods to heal my life and seek out the true magic I have always known was available. More recently, before his passing, I thought I could save him, but I realize he was put on this Earth as my father to save me. I am so grateful to him for giving me my life.

I don't regret the choice I made for myself and what I had to do, because during that time, I was healing my Self, my heart and my mind. Thanks to yoga, all the authors of the various self-help books, my mother, my kids, my husband and Kundalini yoga, I am forever awakening to the Magic instead of remaining a victim of the pain. With this consciousness, I see the other side of pain and understand how to live a magical life. This chiseling of my psyche and renewal of perspective that I work to maintain leads me to experience this one present moment.

It is the present moment that is so magical because all the decisions and events that I chose are the sum total of what I reap today. It is truly a gift that Life is set up in this way for everyone because with some simple practice and a dab of focus, which allows us to become aware of the big picture, we can consciously make choices and decisions in every moment that will shape our destiny; instead of allowing our subconscious mind decide. And the thing is, we all need help awakening. I remember believing years ago that I was aware, but what I am living today is the most sustainably awakened reality. I have always dreamed at the core of my mind about living this way and it continues to improve every day thanks to the secret technology of Kundalini yoga and believing in the Magic of Life. Here is the next meditation to create awareness in your own life.

Meditation:
Become Calm "Earth to Self"

Extend your Jupiter finger (pointer) and lock your thumb over all the other fingers. Find the song "Sat Nam Sat Nam Wahe Guru Wahe Guru" online. Sit with you're your spine straight. Close your eyes and concentrate deeply on the movement.

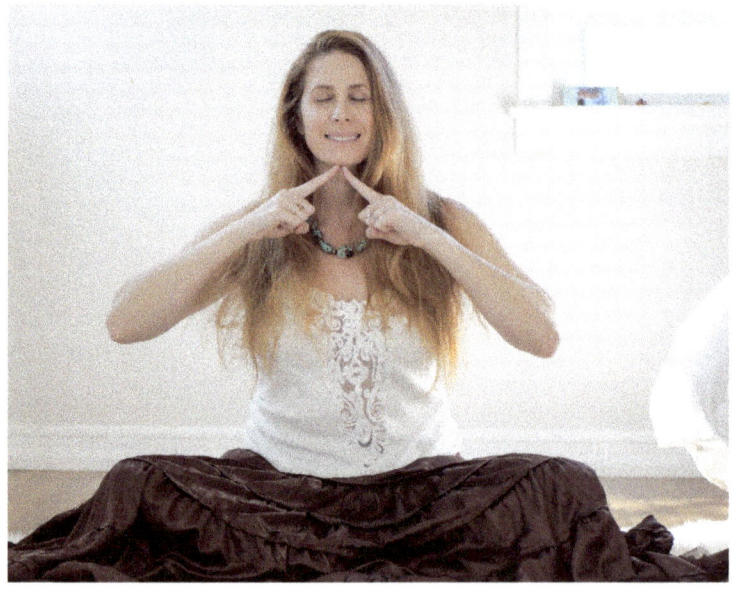

On Sat point your Jupiter fingers toward the floor on either side of you.
On Nam point your pointer fingers towards the middle of your chin.

When you are very tense or confused about your life in the moment, do this to become calm, quiet and peaceful.

Chapter 2

Challenging events ending in Victory

"If you can't fly, then run, if you can't run then walk, if you can't walk then crawl, but whatever you do you have to keep moving forward."

    -Martin Luther King, Jr.

Life gifts us circumstances to challenge us because Life knows that we must grow stronger and become more aligned with our inner self. If you take a moment to ponder, birth is our first life challenge and we all come out crying from that experience. Life knows that we CAN grow and in what way we MUST grow. Therefore, Life tests us. Life knows where we are going and what we need to get there because Life has the GPS.

I have begun to understand, in a subtle way, how our soul remembers what deal it made towards growth before coming back to life. I believe our soul IS what guides us towards the circumstances we NEED in order to acquire a skill or strength for the next level of growth. Our soul literally gave us the perfect mud pond to grow our own lotus flower. Therefore, if we look at all our challenging moments in life as opportunities to evaluate us to the outcomes, instead of remaining stuck in the challenge, we can get through them in a clarified manner. After we're through the challenge, we must measure if we changed, grew or evolved and it is something we measure from the inside.

Growing up, I had a very analytical mind and I still do, hence this book. For example, if something at school, such as a conversation or action I observed happen to me that I was upset about, I would review it over and over all night long so that it would not repeat itself. I remember being so angry with myself for mishandling many situations. Often, I discovered that I failed to use my voice and speak up for myself even after I came to conclusions during my self-analysis. Later in my young adult life as I slowly started to wake up, I would still analyze everything, knowing I had room to improve, but I finally began to test my results and speak up. I believe it was a way to gauge my progress so that I could do better every time. This is a commitment I made after reading the book, "The Fifth Agreement" by Don Miguel Ruiz where he explains not to make assumptions. Instead ask questions that lead to a truth or answer instead of trying to guess about the other person. It was my openness to look within that created something positive and for my growth.

Consequently, I reviewed situations over the years with consistent themes, which proved to me that I was not changing enough. That became frustrating for me because I felt so stuck and so stagnant. I was very impatient with myself, but I did not have any tools how to go faster. Therefore, I remained self critical inside and I made a ton of mistakes. Being so impatient with myself because I desired to advance more quickly actually made me advance slower. The reality of my stagnation became vivid when life felt uncomfortable or my challenge was too big. I have read recently and come to agree that we need to get comfortable being uncomfortable in this life. It requires inner grit, caliber and stamina to remain calm in any situation, but only then will we be at ease. That takes mindfulness, acceptance and patience. Yogi Bhajan said, "Patience pays" and it truly does once we settle into the faith and let go.

Once I began asking and searching for help through the use of self-help books, alternative therapy, podcasts, radio programs, yoga and conversations with wiser people, I began to solidify my method of inner growth. As I said earlier, doing all of this truly taught me how to change from the inside out. I was able to realize most of the uncomfortable occurrences in my life that I could not learn from before, were due to a lack of clear communication towards another or myself. That led me to become more patient with my path, truly let go and live through my process. Upon becoming more patient, I began to see just how much my communication with myself mattered the most in order to change.

From then on, every time an event seemed "bad," it turned out to be quite a useful learning experience for my mind because I could self talk my own way to clarity or mindfulness. Becoming mindful takes the most patience because it must be practiced like a muscle to be made stronger. Plus there are so many layers to our minds, it must be practiced daily and with the science of neuroplasticity, brain grows and we become more aware. Once we peel away one habitual thought we come to the next and then Life will test us to see if we are truly being mindful. It has come to the point in my life where every experience is now something that will help me flex my mindfulness muscle knowing all the while that my inner conversation is most important.

It is a good learning experience to work hard and receive the benefits especially when the inner dialog is positive and motivating. The practice of inner work builds immense character and grit. That is something I only discovered recently in my life. I never liked hard work in my younger life because I thought things should come easy to me and certain things did. I got my first job at Café Montana simply because I was confident I could work there. I got the job as a hostess at fifteen.

After many times of receiving things without any hard work, I realized I was not as fulfilled with what I had received. I also didn't maintain a grateful attitude towards what I was receiving. So, after many years of disappointment, I understood that hard work, patience and perseverance is part of the journey towards joyful and magical fulfillment because we learn to become more grateful with every achievement. Life requires constant grit, excitement and motivation to make the breakthroughs that align with Magic.

Kundalini yoga and power yoga prior, helped me to understand that when we breathe through what is uncomfortable, we can get through any block. Through patience, perseverance and "keeping up" in a Kundalini yoga class or meditation, we break the glass ceiling to get to the next floor. Kundalini yoga puts us in the most uncomfortable situations and our habitual ways of listening to our negative thoughts flare up. The perseverance of "keeping up" in the posture creates a repetition and we begin to uncover our habitual thoughts that hold us back. The neurologist, Dr. Joe Dispenza explains that to "build more positive neuro-pathways we must become less attached to our old habits" in "What the Bleep Do We Know." Kundalini yoga creates the experience of detaching from a negative habitual thought bringing us towards the possibility of creating a new neuro synapse connection and habit.

Most self help people say that when something happens that is positive, we must celebrate by feeling higher vibrations inside. By feeling better more often, we are applying this law of creating new habits in the brain. A byproduct of neurons making new synapses is more positive inner dialog and space to create pathways that we decide to program into the brain. This requires self-awareness and it can begin with a simple ritual of noticing every inner victory of observation, (if you cannot get to a Kundalini yoga class.) A victory on the inside can be noticing a negative habitual thought and turning it to a more supportive thought or simply noticing a habitual pattern. It is the awareness that is something to be celebrated.

In my childhood, I had so few "celebratory" inner moments because I had too many other things I was dealing with, which is what led to my feeling constantly in immense darkness and inner fear. Luckily, I had the Magic of Life on my side because I did have a handful of positive occurrences that I will remember forever. They were placed in my path like one of those treats you land on in the game Candyland. I just happened to land on these particular eye-opening, (or mindfulness opening) experiences that I categorize as synchronistic and magical. I have come to adore and expect sychronicity everyday.

Franklin Elementary School in Santa Monica would throw an amazing Halloween carnival for kids every year; it probably still does. They made it super fun for the students and community by creating a haunted house, games to play using tickets, a cake walk, a costume parade and of course cotton candy. After four years of being a student, I was finally older and able to do more of what I wanted because I got organized in advance. That year, I decided to make a cake to enter into the cakewalk. I had never participated in the cakewalk game in previous years despite the inner urge.

The cakewalk was a game where all the kids who entered had to make a cake decorated with a Halloween theme. The game was to walk in a big circle until the music stopped, similar to musical chairs. When we stopped, we were standing over a number on the ground. Someone would announce a random number and if it was where we were standing, we won the corresponding numbered cake. I spent lots of time decorating my cake to look very spooky and yummy. When I went to the carnival, as I did every year with friends, I was so excited to participate in the cakewalk that I just left my friends; which was super rare for me to only think of myself.

We got to the end of the game where hardly any more cakes were left and suddenly, they called the number I was standing over. When I went to get the corresponding numbered cake, it was so beautiful! It looked better than mine and I was in shock that I had won anything. I went home that afternoon feeling like I had won the lottery and boy did I celebrate that most yummy win. That was a good day.

The next event I can allow myself to be celebrated was much more challenging and uncomfortable. It came a few years later, when I was about to enter high school. My friends and I were all auditioning for the highest dance team at SAMO together. Since I had grown up dancing, I was familiar with dance auditions, but scared nonetheless. They seemed unfair and were stressful for me, but dancing was something I knew deep down that I was good at because I loved to perform dances. The pressure of the audition always gave me a feeling like I couldn't make the cut.

I had previously auditioned for a dance company at eight and nine, but self sabotaged my mind with anxious negative thinking and didn't make it. I auditioned at ten and again didn't make it, all the while watching the company dancers do such amazing dances, dancing in movies, dancing in television and I longed to be in that group. I felt so insecure during those years and despite being apart of middle school drill team, inside I felt like a failure. During middle school, I made the dance team every year, but it wasn't the same to me as the Santa Monica Dance Company.

At my dance school, for those who were in the early days of "the dance company," many went on to do movies, television, or professional musicians. So, at eleven when I finally made it onto senior dance company at Santa Monica dance studio, I felt like I had made it. After two years of dance company and drill team in middle school, I was going to high school. All my friends and I wanted to be on the highest dance team at Samohi called, "Songs." My friends and I all auditioned together, but that day I felt I hadn't done my best. I remember leaving the audition feeling so upset with myself. Almost like I had failed again at something I really wanted.

I went home that day with tears streaming down my face to my mother and sister. I remember making my mother stop the car on the way home because I was so upset with myself. I was having so many habitual negative thoughts of me not being good enough. They were racing through my mind and almost confirming my reason to be upset. I felt like every thought would push me lower and lower into my darkness.

When the list of who made the team went up at the high school, my friends and I went into the counselor's office at our middle school to call the high school. My friends and the counselor picked me to talk on the phone to ask who was on the list. I will never forget hearing my name and NONE of my friends' names. I felt so overwhelmed in that moment with mixed emotions of joy, for myself, and utter fear of announcing the bad news to my friends, that instead of telling them the truth, I lied.

I told my three best friends that they had all made it onto the Songs team and I had not. Needless to say, I was in the most magical kind of shock imaginable, but I lost all three of my "best" friends. I realized that I had triumphed for something that I truly wished for and thought I wouldn't obtain. All my sadness and darkness the day of the audition pushed me to a point of truly letting go of the outcome, since I was sure I had not succeeded. The universe knew I had worked for years to be a better dancer and the Magic of Life decided to reward me as a big surprise.

Unfortunately, because of my fear of hurting my friend's feelings and not taking responsibility with confidence to tell them the truth, I had not triumphed with my friendships. One of my best friends had made it onto senior dance company at Santa Monica dance center a year before me and I was always so jealous of her, until I made it onto Songs and she did not. All these years later, I am still grateful for the successes and the challenges that I faced in my difficult teenage years, even the ones where I lost girlfriends. As it is said, "friends are like stars they come and go, but the ones that stay are the ones that glow." I still find that girls/women are the most challenging of life's color palette for self-growth in relationships because we are so complicated when we are stuck to our feelings. Female relationships, whether it is with my own sisters, mother, mother-in-law or girl friends, are so tricky and my relationships with girls and women over the years have been a point of pain for me.

We women have so many complicated feelings. We are capable of so much in the home and workplace, yet we have much to still learn in our intimate relationships. It is difficult to understand how to handle our emotions because we believe we are our emotions and we become so consumed in those feelings. Remaining in the hamster wheel of feelings can push the best of us to make isolating decisions as I have done many times. Ideally, we must instead try to make honest, expansive and supportive decisions for the benefit of all humans so that we are not storing hurt for later or being stuck in low vibratory frequencies. Yogi Bhajan said, "Our issues are in our tissues" meaning all our stored pain from our lives get stuck in our bodies because we weren't honest with our selves first, or our friends, families, colleagues, teachers and others.

      Is it surprising to me that breast cancer is almost the leading cancer women develop? We women could learn to be a bit more like men when it comes to communication because, as I watch my two boys when they have a problem, they say it to each other then it is handled. Depending on the type of relationship it is between women, to simply let out how we are feeling when we are feeling it could be healing for both parties and it feels highly transparent. That way we are truly taking care of our feelings as a first step towards the growth of the relationship. This will lead to more responsibility towards improving our awareness. This is important for the energy to not stagnate in our tissues. It is important for women to support other women, instead of getting even or being vengeful, but it takes total awakening from within to get past all those lower frequency emotions such as jealousy, envy, fear, sadness, grudges, pain and hate. In the new paradigm, women must support other women.

      The most intense challenge that life sent my way and one that I define as feeling the most abysmal of my young adult life was suicide. Suicide was a challenging concept and recurring thought for me all of high school and into college. I believe it was due to the toll that unconsciousness played on me when girls were just being girls, but also it was about my misunderstanding of my own childhood and the effect it had on me. The last time I thought I wanted to commit suicide was into my second year of college. I left my college in an all girls private school in Columbia, Missouri after the first year to come back home to California.

My experience at the girl's school supported my sub-consciously programmed feeling that women were not to be trusted. I had a roommate who I became very close with the first semester at school, but after thanksgiving that friendship quickly went south. She and I had joined the same sorority, I had gone to her house multiple times and we did everything together. It was so fun until it wasn't. Second semester it became so bad, I made her move out of our dorm room because she was so passive aggressive towards me. All the other girls in the dorm we were friends with took sides. I still don't know what happened with her.

It made me stronger in some ways to kick her out of our dorm room and weaker in others, but it got me to move forward with my life. I had been working at Gap Kids and finished out the year in peace, but unfortunately I decided to quit that school and the full scholarship I had to their theatre program. I felt so done that I didn't even stay for summer stock, which turned out to be a big learning experience. As soon as I got home from that year I decided to take a semester off and just work. At Gap kids, I felt confident with my ability to do well at work. I loved working there because it was the biggest Gap in Santa Monica and lots of celebrities came in to buy their kids clothes. Not only that, but I loved my managers and the work I got to do.

Summer had passed and it was the Fall semester I took a break from College. I began an acting school in NoHo where Jeff Goldblum taught and I thought it would be good for my acting career to be in the "real" business instead of learning theatre at school. So, I continued working at Gap Kids and I was moving forward, but still having trouble with my mind's habit of negative thoughts. Then, I began a homeopathic remedy treatment thanks to a magical healing session I had with an Indian woman named, Gaya. She said that I had darkness and I, of course agreed. My inner world of the darkness was over powering my light. I explained to her that I considered multiple times to commit suicide because I wanted so badly to have more light than dark. Then, one day on my lunch break at Gap Kids, I finally wanted to give up.

I went to jump off a cliff that overlooked the beach and the Palisades. It was right where hundreds of people run two different flights of stairs. I was looking over the cliff and I felt such a darkness looming over any positive horizons I might foresee. I was stuck in my negative mind and blaming my challenging beginning for being so stuck. After my female friendships were lost and my boyfriend wasn't someone I really felt good being with, I couldn't get my mind to be positive. As I was analyzing everything, it became too overwhelming for me and decided to jump to end it all.

At that very moment, I stood up on the cliff and I promise you as I was about to jump something shook me backwards. It wasn't an invisible energy as strong as in my story from the beginning of this book, but it was subtle and it woke me up. I realized I was not going to end my life that day or ever. I decided I would get help in a new way than I had ever done before. That small synchronistic sign helped me to grasp onto my inner light and change my life. The next couple of months that followed, I found my yoga guru in Bryan Kest and I began trying more homeopathic remedies for depression.

That experience was a wake up call to my way of feeling about myself at that time. I didn't communicate nicely towards myself because I was overly critical instead of being motivational. The small amount of light within me was ignited and began to build over time through small victories scattered throughout my life. Not until that day did I realize that my inner light was not enough to cut out the darkness completely at that young age. I needed more help to have more victories.

I needed more experience, more awakening and more life challenges to get myself to a constant decision of choosing to love myself so much that no darkness overpower the thinking inside of me. I was perhaps a little broken, but in my heart I knew I could become fixed, even without knowing how. It didn't matter how long it would take because getting myself to a place where positivity would lead my life was my ultimate goal. The heart knows what our soul's truth is and the head takes a lot longer.

My inner belief towards self-love was stronger than I could have imagined at that dark time in my life. This inner love must take over for the head and the ego. It is simply the only way we as humans can triumph together in all our lives. It is this ability to see that love is the highest frequency feeling. Love must be our driving force to move towards the paradigm shift for the human race today; where love comes out of our hearts and leads us to our health. If I am able to see the magic that life is full of, then, everyone can and will once we all believe.

Meditation:

Conquer Inner Anger and Burn It Out

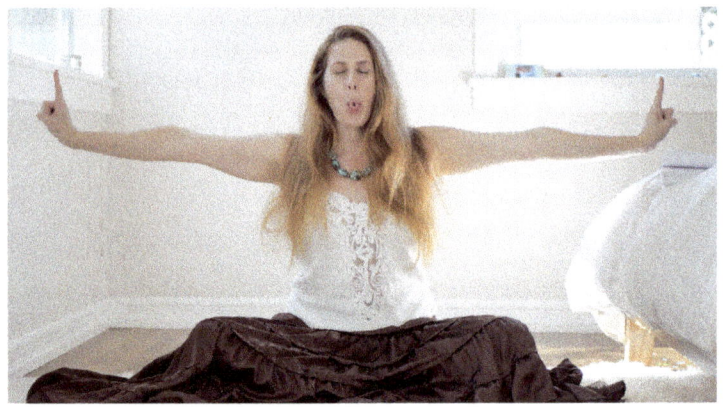

Sit in easy pose with your arms stretched out to the sides.

Jupiter finger points upward stiffly with thumbs locking down all other fingers.

Close your eyes and concentrate on your spine.

Inhale deeply through rolled tongue and exhale through nose.

11 minutes

Finish by inhaling deeply and maintaining the breath for 10 seconds while you. Stretch your arms out strongly. Exhale and repeat this sequence 2 more times.

This meditation can be done either in the morning or in the evening. If you do this every day for 11 minutes, your entire life will change. Do it for 40 days, it will change you personally from A to Z.

Chapter 3

France: "C'est ma vie"

"In what country on earth would you rather live" He answered, "Certainly in my own where are all my friends my relations and the earliest and sweetest affections and recollections of my life." "Which would be your second choice" his answer "France."

-Thomas Jefferson

I have an addiction to airplane flying because of the excitement of the beginning of an adventure towards something new just beyond my horizon. My cells come to attention and scintillate knowing that from the moment I step into the airplane, new impossible things are going to happen. I am out of my daily routine and comfort zone. I am preparing myself to be open to the new. The biggest excitement before a new adventure is visiting an unknown location. The idea fills me up with such wonderment, that I begin to feel like I could be going to another galaxy. I imagine how my destination will look, smell, feel and sound. This way of thinking developed over time, but the first time I remember feeling this new wave of creativity, I was fourteen.

It was the trip of my dreams and the first trans-Atlantic flight of my life. I was with my stepsister and stepbrother, but no parents. When we stepped on the plane I did feel butterflies, but the stewardess came to greet us and she told us she was available all the way to Paris if we needed anything. She gave us a necklace that said unaccompanied minor with games and our paperwork inside. We were independent which suited me just fine. When we arrived in Paris, the adventure I had been imagining commenced.

My year and a half of French language lessons at school were about to pay off. People began saying the words I'd learned, "bonjour, comment allez-vous?" Then, when the same people understood what I was saying and responded back to me, I had butterflies of excitement and bubbling achievement in my belly. Even though, I had no idea what they were saying back, I was doing something completely new all by myself. The stewardess took us to a special holding area to wait for the next flight going to Nice. My sister and brother had done it before so, I trusted everything to be fine and go with the flow.

Upon arrival in Nice, I walked out of the terminal with my stepbrother, stepsister, and step grandparents into a different world. Outside, I was infused with the odor of the South of France; a mixture of heat, the Mediterranean Sea, diesel, baguette, cheese, and wine. It was nothing I'd ever experienced and it was potent. The overwhelming feeling of joy hit me like lightening. I was in the zone and ready for this experience.

Arriving at their vineyard was surprising as the smells became more compelling and my perspective of life was expanding by the second. There are speed junkies, adrenaline junkies, and I was quickly becoming a traveling junkie. The bedroom I was introduced to was unlike anything I'd ever seen in my entire life; not even in films. My room had a sink inside and so did my sister and brother's. The toilet was in a tiny room by itself. "Does France not have showers," I thought. Then, I was introduced to the bathroom across the hall with a shower and no toilet. How strange everything is in a different country.

After the acceptance that I was no longer in California hit, I fell asleep after brushing my teeth in my bedroom. When morning came and I went downstairs, I practiced my "Bonjour" and "oui, merci, j'ai bien dormi." I was introduced to an outside terrace overlooking the vineyard with a table made of an old stone olive oil grinding mill. It had huge porous holes all over the top, sides and bottom from the grinding of the olives. Back then the top of the table was not flat and things would fall into the holes, but it was authentic and so French. On the table was a paper bag full of croissants, different kinds of jellies, and yogurts. I felt like I was in heaven at the sight of the table.

My step grandmother, whom I hadn't met before this trip, brings out a gigantic mug and saucer and tells me that my brother and sister always drink hot chocolate for breakfast. I gladly take the grandmother size mug of hot chocolate and my first French croissant. Upon my first bite the fact that I was in France, the land of butter and cheese, sank in. This croissant was the best tasting piece of food I'd ever tasted in my life. I thought croissants in Los Angeles were pretty good, but this was a piece of heaven.

When my brother and sister finally woke up they ran downstairs and began to fight over the rest of the croissants. I had eaten two they were so good, but my brother had three in his hands before our grandmother even brought out their hot chocolates. My sister was fighting with our brother over the fourth croissant in a tug of war type of struggle. I understood how they felt, as I wanted to eat the whole bag, too, when I saw it, but eyes are always larger than stomachs.

That first day we went to a beach, called "Maison Bambou" and it felt like it took forever to get to, but now I realize I was being introduced to the Cote d'Azur traffic. The water was a color of blue I had only seen in the first Blue Lagoon movie. The sand didn't take ten minutes to cross like in Santa Monica; it was like two hops from the car. We were at a restaurant on the beach with rows upon rows of lounge chairs and tan women and men in the most beautiful bathing suits and clothes I'd ever seen. It was like a living magazine.

Our drink cups had a green sugared rim and tasted better than sugar. A jus d'orange or grenadine-a-l'eau was so pretty with the green rim. Lunch proceeded to impress me to an even higher level of satisfaction. Confirming to myself that I was most definitely in heaven. I didn't even like tomatoes before I tried a "tomate mozzarella." Then we had giant shrimp called, gambas, which I had to break open myself. It was the first time I saw an actual full animal on my plate eyes and all. Dessert was ice cream with strawberries and raspberries and I was hooked. I love the Côte d'Azur!

After a week of going to different beach restaurants and eating over a hundred croissants, our grandparents introduced us to, Luna Park, a mini amusement park for kids with a fun house, rides, and above all gummy candy. It was not just any gummy candy, but a table of gummy candy the size of three cafeteria tables. There were gummy sharks, cokes, snakes, cherries, strawberries, eggs, Smurfs, bugs, lips, and of course gummy bears and this was before Sweet Factory type of candy store. The following month in France if there was ever any fighting, it was over whose gummy candy bag had more gummies.

A couple of weeks later I had had enough. The high life was enough and I missed my mom, friends, and dance camp. My imagination began to run wild and I tried to convince my twelve-year old stepsister to run off to Paris. That didn't work so well as we were way too young. I began having asthma attacks and complaining. I forgot that I was still on a joyful adventure. After the month of France was finally over, I was so happy to be going home and to be getting out of this small village that I told myself, "I never want to go back."

I am now forty, I married a French man on my grandparents vineyard, my kids were both born in France and we have lived on the Cote d'Azur for seven years. Little did I know at fourteen, that my love affair with France was just setting into motion. It was not until the moment I got back that I realized just how much fun I'd had in France. Not to mention, I had a killer tan and had lost weight eating croissants and gummy candy. To say it was a memorable experience is an understatement.

The second time I went to France, I was eighteen. This time with the whole family, including the new addition, a baby girl my parents conceived one year before who I had the honor of naming. I was able to see her come into this world through my mother. It was a true miracle. That was the day I saw my stepfather with the same reaction as my own; we both cried with uncontrollable joy. I have carried that bond with me a ever since…(just more of the magic.)

That summer with my family, filled me up with such a complete feeling of true family for the first time. It was something I had been wishing for my entire life and it was the Infinite Divine Source's way of showing me that magic is a certainty. That occasion was imprinted in my psyche as a repair to my difficult beginning. Our family had been reconstructed by my mother, my stepfather and the Magic of Life, which pushed all of us into this life circumstance for our growth. This memory helped me on my journey to becoming more positive.

That trip solidified my interest in French language, as a culture and even part of my destiny. I would continue to visit France often after that, going back alone, with family and even a boyfriend. I continued taking French every year at University because I was determined to speak well. Even after studying French every year in school since seventh grade and visiting France often, I wasn't fluent a year before college graduation. Therefore, Christmas of senior year at University, I decided to go to France for summer to work and get closer to fluency.

It was that summer I truly learned to speak French and it was also that summer that I met my future husband. My grand parents wine was sold at many beach restaurants along the Côte d'Azur. One of the clients and friend of my grandparents with a private beach club had known my grandfather many years. His beach club was called, Maison Bambou and it has since closed. He gave me a night job at his beach club restaurant that prepared Thai food at night and local cuisine during the day. My day job was the same as my stepsister's. We modeled bathing suits at another beach club's boutique.

On my first night at the Thai beach club restaurant, my whole family came to see how the American girl would do on her first night at work in France. It was super fun because our uncle had just been married and everyone from my family came to eat. My job was to ask the orders and serve bottled water, wine and dessert. The water was easy because it had a twist off top, but because it was summer and in France if you're at a private beach club, you're drinking a lot of bottled water due to the heat. The wine was super fun because it was my family's wine, but opening over a hundred wine bottles a night for two months was definitely work.

I learned fast which kind of wine opener was the best and how to open a bottle of wine the French way. You must open it without making too much noise upon pulling the cork out and you must ask who wants to taste the wine to make sure it has not turned. My favorite part was to smell the cork after pulling it out of the bottle and just by the smell I could say whether the bottle was bad or good. It just so happened that the first night, when I had to retrieve the wine, I went to the cute bar tender. The Magic was hinting at something Karmic with this bar tender.

As a side note, I had already visited the beach club several times before my first night to work there and I had already noticed that bar tender. When he introduced himself to me that first night at work, it was by surprise. He caught me towards the end of the night, as I was getting ready to leave. I had plans with my sister and brother to go out on Cote d'Azur to the clubs. He asked me to stay after work to "hang out" and maybe smoke some pot, but I knew I was going out with my sister and brother.

The next night after work, he cornered me and explained that since I had not come the night before, I had to join him that night. When I arrived at his beach bungalow, which was fifty feet away from the restaurant, our boss was there with another female employee. When I saw her, my heart sank a little because I thought the bar tender and her were a couple and since she was also invited I convinced myself they were together. To say that I was intimidated would be exact, because not only was I rusty at understanding French, but speaking French and following a conversation among multiple people is an additional challenge and everyone there was smoking pot.

I had done my fair share of pot smoking, having been to Amsterdam and growing up in Santa Monica, but it was not something I wanted to do the first night I presented myself. I tried to join in as best I could by smoking pot and pretending to understand their conversation in French. I felt like I was in the scene from the film, Last of the Mohicans where everyone is speaking in a different language and as the man sits long enough, he begins to resonate with the vibration and finally understands what is being said. Every moment that passed, I became less and less excited about my hopes of having a conversation with the bar tender. Plus my grandparents and my parents were waiting at home for me to arrive after work. During the summer months on Cote d'Azur there are drunk driving accidents everyday.

It got later and later and I needed to leave, but right at the moment I wanted to stand up, I physically could not get up between the fatigue of my new job and the pot. The next second after my thought, my boss said he was going home. I thought to myself, "me too," but I could not remember the words to say in French. When he left and it was only myself there with the bar tender and the other girl I thought, "say good night." We continued to talk a few more minutes and when I finally decided how to say, "I have to leave" and thank them for the invitation, the girl took the words out of my mouth and quickly left.

Finally, the bar tender and I were the only two people, but what was I supposed to say being so nervous and inapt in French? He must have felt the same way because in the next few moments he kissed me. The next morning I woke up to Mika asking me if he could make me breakfast or something to drink. I responded with about the only thing I remembered at that moment of shock, "chocolat chaud, s'il vous plait." He brought me a tray with hot chocolate and a croissant. He was so sweet to be taking care of me like that the morning after our first night together, that was not something I was used to in the least, but it was something I was ready to receive. Twenty minutes later, I found out my grandparents had called the police and hospitals looking for me and I was in big trouble.

Mika became my French teacher because he didn't speak English hardly at all and he would correct me all summer long. It turns out, the French are extremely tight assed about their precious language, but making all those mistakes is what helped me to learn. I stayed with him for the rest of the summer in that beach bungalow listening to the waves every morning and every night. My set up felt so magical and I was having so much fun bouncing between the woods of the vineyard to the beach it didn't matter if I didn't understand every conversation. I felt happy. Somehow we were able to communicate despite my broken French. He told me years later that my accent was charming and how I would constantly make little mistakes with masculine and feminine certainly made him laugh.

Learning French thoroughly taught me more about my own mother tongue of English. I never felt I did well in grammar at school and learning French forced me to understand grammar in language. I became fascinated in how language began at the beginning with languages like Sanskrit, Aramaic or any archaic language by the root of words and where they come from. English is Germanic, which is an Indo-European language with roots in Sanskrit unlike French, Spanish, and Portuguese, which are based in Latin or Phoenician before that. This intrigued me to understand whom people are within their culture based on the language they speak and where that symbology comes from. Daydreaming of this was easy as I was studying the culture in France on a daily basis.

Meeting at the Thai restaurant on the beach in France was an easy bridge to walk over because the French who owned the Thai restaurant had homes in Thailand. A year after I met Mika, we found ourselves learning Thai together in Thailand. Thai is similar to Chinese as it has a tonal alphabet, but it is not characterized as a written language earlier than Latin and Sanskrit. Although the Ancient Chinese do have a written history dated to five thousand years. I began learning Thai quite easily and understood that I really have an interest and a knack for learning languages. My destiny led me to France and France opened my life up to the rest of the world.

Since 2000 when I met Mika to the present day, I lived on and off in France, New York and Los Angeles. In that time space, Mika and I broke up five times, got back together six times, moved four times, got married, and birthed two boys. The longest I went without seeing him was a year and a half. The longest I went without seeing my family was the same. Being away from those we love, teaches us to appreciate them in a deep way; no matter how angry or frustrated we may feel around them.

It is during the time away from my family and my country that I developed my own new identity independent of my prior identity. I believe leaving my family and friends forced me to really look at myself and become best friends with myself over the years. When there are no more distractions or people relying on your identity, an opportunity to re-invent or better oneself becomes a possibility and desire. In France I felt so free to explore myself and Life, not only did I learn more about my true self but, I learned how to cook from scratch, I learned how to work hard, I learned about the EU government, I learned how that I could have a new perspective. I was standing in the energy of that culture of French fashion, French food, French thinking simply being an expat. That is what I had to do because I had to adapt to France.

Leaving America for that long was very challenging for my old ways and thoughts, but I really grew into my self-confidence.

Some people never leave their family's side during their whole lifetime and it can be a very secure feeling. They grow up in the same town or city together with siblings, cousins, aunts and uncles. The kids go to school together and the parents stay friends with one another. Barbeques are frequent and life is simple in the community setting, but of course the minute there is a problem, the whole family is aware and involved. There are many families in France like that, including my husband's.

His mother lived next door to all her sisters and brother almost all of her young adult life. Mika grew up next to his family, playing with his cousins and hardly has any friends who aren't family. His mother still lives next door to her sister and their mother. Their family is extremely close and they rely on each other for everything. Most of France is like that. The families grow and evolve at the same rate, but now with technology and easy travel the younger generations are have started exploring outside of their family comfort zone. Those younger generations are pushing the family to embrace a global reality.

I didn't grow up living next to my mother's family. She decided to live far away from her parents, sisters, and brother. We always kept in touch with our family over the phone and almost visited annually, but it was not the same as having cousins at the same school. In a way, it forced us to make friends and create a new family, a family of our own choosing. Consequently, we were also fortunate to not have familial traditions and expectations placed on us. We could explore new religions, philosophy's, try new things to create new traditions and my mother did somewhat engage in exploration, but never adopted any new ways of ritual or tradition. I am nonetheless grateful for my life not being ordinary because I was able to live a myriad of experiences, which helped me to grow.

    Among all the experiences France and its' tangents brought into my life, my step-father, my husband, language, culture, wine, cheese, croissants, holidays, government and all the gifts, the most incredible experience remains who it has carved me into today. Being shaped by many cultures is conducive to having tolerance, acceptance and compassion for life and humanity. If we are so lucky to have a life situation or a daily practice that teaches us to create clarity of perspective, we can learn to see our future destiny being chiseled one piece at a time and we can walk proudly through our days towards that destiny. We can feel the magic of life lifting us up higher and higher to our full potentials. Experience takes time.

Meditation:

Correct The Five Tattwas

Sit in easy pose with elbows bent and palms facing each other at should height.

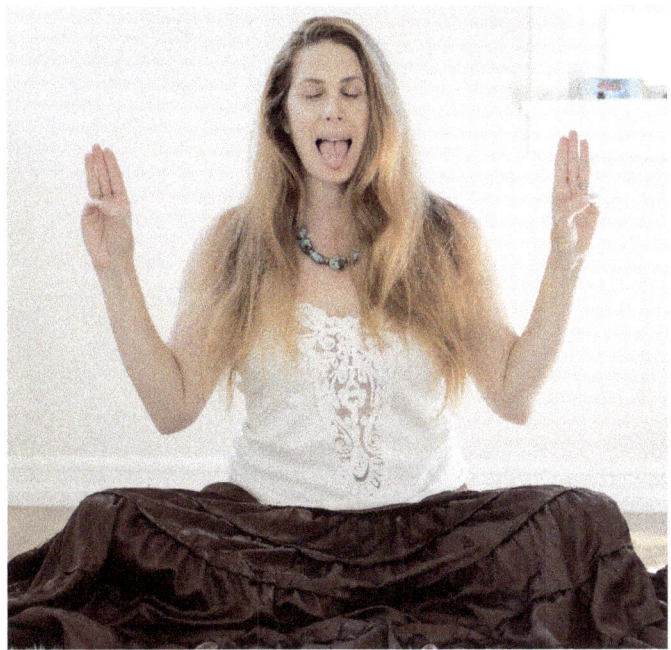

Touch the tip of Mercury finger to tip of thumb and keep the other three fingers straight up. Stick the tongue all the way out and breath in and out fast through the mouth called dog breath from the diaphragm.

10 minutes

Finish and inhale deeply, roll your tongue inward to maintain your breath for 15 seconds. Exhale and repeat 2 more times. This kriya unlocks the diaphragm, takes away anger and can return your to the innocent state of childhood.

Chapter 4

Yoga, Yogic philosophy and me

"Yoga is not about touching your toes, it is what you learn on the way down."
-Jigar Gor

"Yoga is not about self improvement, it's about self-acceptance."
 - Gurmukh Kaur Khalsa

"I have been a seeker and I still am, but I stopped asking the books and the stars. I started listening to the teaching of my Soul."
 -Rumi

A journey is meant to be long, adventurous, challenging, beautiful and in the end satisfying. We must get from the beginning to the end but, along the way, our journey stays interesting and keeps us on our toes. It can be perceived this way because if we have a mission that we focus on with our full concentration, we stay in it. We have all had the experience of going on a trip, only to learn of unplanned challenges such as traffic, flat tires or delayed flights. Do we become angry, shout profanities, complain and cry? Of course we do; we do that because we have forgotten about the adventurous spirit during the challenges, but we are always so happy once we arrive.

Life is the journey of the soul and we forget that because we are always striving towards possessions, arrival and control. I have heard it said many times lately that, when we arrive on our deathbed, we cannot take our family, our possessions nor our money with us. If we believe this to be true and think about it for a minute, why do we spend so much time slowly killing ourselves to have money, control and possessions? I understand that where our society is in this linear time continuum, we use paper money to acquire things of comfort and luxury, we compete to succeed and we dream industrious dreams. The fact is money and possessions are an illusion and a distraction to where the real show is, inside all of us. We continued to believe we must look outside to society, to culture, to priests, rabbis, parents, presidents and anyone else, instead of looking within for our answers. With the new paradigm, all of this has shifted.

Yoga is the outwardly practice for the body to learn to look inside by feeling. When we are doing yoga, we cannot be experiencing our outward luxuries or our worries for the yoga to heal us. It is impossible to be on a yoga mat and in our rat wheel competing to succeed or else we will get hurt. It is designed to gets us out of our heads even for just a few minutes. We have a person suggesting movements to us for an hour or more and during that time we are asked to do different things with our physical bodies. The most important of which is to breathe. I love yoga! I have loved it in previous lifetimes and in this lifetime. I have loved it since I was sixteen years old when I tried it for the first time. All of my years of dancing prepared my body to be good at classical yoga like Hatha or Ashtanga because of the strength and flexibility they procure. Yoga was the perfect alternative to dance class, which is what I grew up doing. Yoga focused on the physical body being a bridge from the inner world to the outer world. Through twenty years of yoga, I healed my mind more as a by-product to all the damage classical dancing caused to my mind.

    My first yoga class was at Yogaworks on Montana. I remember the woman teaching me about holding my arms a certain way and squaring my hips while holding a warrior pose. My body had never been placed in a position like that in a dance class and yet, I felt so at home. It was so hard to hold, but felt so good on a deeper more subtle level, almost as if my body had needed this my whole life. I pushed my body, I held strong while releasing tension and I learned to breathe. Finally, at the end when we had to rest, I felt amazing. I was in love with yoga.

    I continued this type of yoga a few times a month for the rest of that year. Then, junior year of high school my boyfriend's mother and I talked about yoga. She took me to my first Kundalini class. She was very into it and wanted to introduce me to a different kind of yoga. It was Kundalini yoga at the Hare Krishna temple in Culver City. Almost everyone in class was wearing light orange clothes and doing a form of Hatha yoga that was fast and difficult. They were chanting, but there was little to no explanation and it did not feel welcoming. I left that class thinking I would never do that kind of yoga again, but what I failed to see was that destiny knocking on my door.

My yogic journey pushed me further along the path and my senior year of high school, I ran into a friend a year older who did yoga. He and I shared stories about our various yoga experiences and his sounded intriguing. He practiced Power yoga with a man named Bryan Kest and he told me to come try sometime. I thought that since I had been going to Yogaworks and I felt like I knew what I was doing and I could join him one time. I had been experiencing an inner feeling of wanting more experiences with other forms of yoga at that point anyway. So, I went with him to one of Bryan's power yoga classes the very next week.

Finding Power yoga with Bryan Kest at nineteen turned out to be the biggest blessing of my life. I quickly fell in love with it, but not because he had a line out the door and down the street because it resonated deep inside, like a remembering. What I saw first surprised and intimidated me to see so many people. I quickly found my friend in line and I waited with him to go into the upstairs room. There was a subtle excitement in the energy of the people waiting; like when you are about to go into a concert. When we got inside, the room was huge and everyone was setting up their yoga mats closely to one another in rows. The room was slightly steamy and warm. The street outside was audible, but the excitement inside had much more movement. People were visiting with their friends across the room, going to the bathroom, and talking to the teacher off to the side in this energetic excited manner that was contagious. Once everyone was set up with the mats lain down, Bryan announced we were to begin shortly. The minute he started talking is when I fell in love with Power yoga.

Bryan had an assuring voice that put one at ease right away, all while being present in a way that felt palpable, speaking interconnectedly and human at the same time. His explanations to begin the class were so well described and his words were simple and direct like a guided meditation to reach into the humanity inside of us. His street talk style of relating to everyone by using examples from our collective Los Angeles lives was his way to get us ready to do some seriously challenging yoga.

In Bryan's class I developed an experience of my body unlike any other kind of exercise ever before. I went everyday for at least two years because it was so exciting to feel that good. I was awakening and evolving my mind and my body fast. My physical body was the strongest and healthiest it ever had been before. After doing yoga either in Bryan's class or at home for three plus years, I became devoted. I began doing it on vacation and teaching my friends. I went to Cabo San Lucas with two girlfriends when I was twenty-one and on that vacation, I remember teaching them power yoga in the stairwell of our hotel. I was focused on creating a daily practice of self-discipline in yoga.

The social stigma of having a healthy thin body at twenty-one, especially in Los Angeles was my impetus for a daily practice, but my mind began to notice a clear subtle benefit, too. It was like I could see my thoughts more clearly, I was becoming un-attached to them and I was less disturbed by them. That is when I realized yoga is a true self-healing practice. I began to do something new with my thoughts. The negative depressing dark thoughts ceased to affect me in the same toll. The moments of challenge in my journey stopped making me react with profanities or frustration towards myself. I was beginning to experience Niyama, Pratyahara and Dharana, which are built into Patanjali's eight limbs of Ashtanga yoga. Around that time, a friend of mine Julia, from acting class invited me to a Kundalini class. I did not know what to expect after having had that experience years before that I wasn't fond to remember.

It was a woman named Gurmukh Kaur Khalsa and she was a sikh. There were lots of people at her house who were Sikhs, too, but there were also people there who were not as well. We all gathered on the floor in her living room. I was next to Julia and all I remember was doing really hard arm movements for what seemed like an hour. I couldn't keep my arms up and all the people there were so focused and immersed, but I couldn't keep my focus. Then, we began chanting and singing, which again felt extremely odd to me. Overall, I was again having a hard time at her house.

After the class, a vegetarian meal was provided and everyone was so nice. I spoke with Gurmukh, but at twenty-one I was not confident enough to express the difficulty I experienced during the Kundalini yoga. I was still too young, embarrassed and attached to my ego. Therefore, I could not ask her advice for what I truly may have needed at that time, which was to keep up with Kundalini. As we journey through our lives, we are on a specific path for a specific reason and sometimes we can advance quickly, if we are very self motivated but, most of the time we choose to experience challenges over and over to help us grow. If we are not aware of our cycles of repetitive experiences, we will stay stuck. I went back to her house two or three more times, mostly for the vegetarian dinners, but in the end, I decided to continue on my power yoga journey.

After two more years of daily practicing and experiencing ups and downs in life, I began teaching Bryan Kest's power yoga. I got my first job teaching power yoga at a local private gym and I gave all I could to my students as I had learned. It felt so right and invigorating to teach something I was so passionate about. I remember teaching my students similarly to how Bryan would; explaining about life and the breath being so important. I remember having an easy time teaching and really loving it. Many of my students would come talk to me after class and tell me how good they felt, different stories of benefit they experienced in their lives and/or to ask questions. Then, I announced I was leaving the private gym to go live with my French boyfriend in France and my students were very upset.

Upon arrival in France, I quickly decided to continue teaching yoga, but this time privately at various five star hotels on the Côte d'Azur. There were no yoga studios and the French yoga community was small. Therefore, I did what everyone in the area did and I taught for the tourists. I met many upscale people from all over the world, many of them famous or rich enough to stay at the five star hotels and pay for private yoga classes. It was a good way to make money at that time while I was figuring my life out.

As the years past and I moved around a lot, teaching yoga stayed the staple back burner job. I taught private yoga in New York City at Equinox and taught group classes in a small ahead of its' time yoga, oxygen bar, massage and juice bar. Then, over the years wherever I was living at the moment, I would teach privates whether in France or Los Angeles. I even taught an Arabian princess for a week at Casa Del Mar in Santa Monica and a celebrity at the Peninsula Hotel in Beverly Hills, but I still was not seeing any role models of yoga teachers making this their career. The magic of life was still a desire, but the alignment within the belief was not in my field of vision. I was lost.

I continued teaching private yoga this way and practicing on my own, but I wasn't completely drug free yet, which is one important rubric of yoga. Yoga is about being able to handle life with equanimity and drugs shift the chemicals in the body to be unbalanced. Meaning, without being drug free we continue reacting to every little thing that challenges us on our path no matter how much yoga. What I did not realize at that time was that, yoga is a scientific technology and if used fully, can be a tool to elevate our Self and our life. I was strong in my physical body and becoming stronger in my mental body, but I was not meditating, which is also a rubric of yoga. If we remain a person who dabbles in many things instead of having confidence to go completely into something, we cannot reap the deepest rewards available. Yoga is the science of life and one cannot dabble in truth; one must life truth.

I realize now the journey in my twenties was twisted with many turns and my subconscious programming was leading me, instead of my highest consciousness. Although I learned how to stay calm and breathe in major life situations, I was not aware enough. Yoga is not only about the asanas. It is about the entire life of the individual. When done correctly, the practitioner includes meditation and a deep awareness of everything inside and outside, seen and unseen. This chapter is about yoga, but all life experiences functioned together with ebb and flow of my practice. Early in my growth, I was leading a life in crisis. Being stuck in the program of always looking for "real" jobs or having an "acceptable career" was distracting me from my inner self and all the possibility available to change. Instead, if perhaps I had gotten into Kundalini yoga and meditation at Gurmukh's house, I would have strengthened my mind, body, soul, soul connection, spirit, awareness and self-confidence. Unfortunately, my free will chose to experience many different really hard things and didn't lead me to Kundalini until later. Of course looking back, I know that I was on the perfect path for me throughout this entire time and I would not change it in the slightest. It was a confusing time, the Piscean Age.

At first, I did interior design for a few years at California Closets. Then after I got married, I still wanted to be in the entertainment industry so I tried being a director and went to New York Film Academy for directing and producing film. Following school, I produced a commercial in France for my family's vineyard. It came out great and I paid off my college debt, but it didn't fulfill me on a soul level, plus it was a lot of work all by myself. I still hadn't reached the level realizing my purpose with an inner drive full of passion, grit, self-understanding or self-confidence to make a career out of directing, acting, interior design, or teaching yoga.

In 2009, life gave me another special gift in the form of a huge challenge. I had been married a year and we got pregnant on our first real try. I had been doing prenatal yoga for three and a half months with a local Hatha and birth preparation teacher and all the other mothers loved it as much as me. The challenge Life gifted me with was unfortunate because at seventeen weeks, we learned I had to have an abortion. The baby, Grace as per my biological father, had a rare form of Down's Syndrome. The doctors told my husband and I that she was not well enough to live through until birth. This was a crisis that Power yoga could not get me through. I was hardly given the choice to keep her or abort and suddenly she was gone. That was the darkest, saddest and lowest point of my married life. I remember needing to turn more deeply into yogic and spiritual thinking after that, but Hatha and Power yoga were falling short for the depth of my pain.

I began to deeply immerse myself into many self-help writers and healers, reading all the self-help books I could find. If someone told me about a good book on connecting deeper, I would read or listen to the authors speak. Through climbing up the ladder process, I put my faith into the Magic of life without telling anyone because I felt it was my only choice for sanity. I knew my purpose of wanting to experience being a mother would arrive. I was determined to have children because I knew it was part of my purpose and immediately that became my mission.

Finally in 2012, after many miscarriages, many new methods of creating new beliefs to adopt and medical tests, we decided, with the immense support of a French Fertility doctor to do IVF. I was working with a wonderful French fertility clinic and my doctor knew what she was doing. Fortunately, it worked on the first time and deep inside I felt that my commitment to believe in the Magic on a subtle slow level began to truly function. I received a lovely Sagittarian birthday present to end my year and I became pregnant with a healthy baby boy. My wish had come true and my destiny began. The only caveat and challenge was that I was in France and not in Los Angeles surrounded by family, but even this turned into a blessing in disguise.

My lovely mother knew how sad I was not to have family and friends around me during that special time. So, she encouraged me to go find prenatal yoga somewhere around where I lived. Even after I assured her there was none, she insisted. Moreover, I had done prenatal yoga in Los Angeles during my first pregnancy with my daughter, before I was forced to abort, and that did not end well. Needless to say, I was not enthusiastic about prenatal yoga in France at all, which was a mistake for feeling the scar upon my heart would not heal.

Despite my reluctance, my mom went online and found a local prenatal yoga class down the road from me. After the New Year, I went to my first class and it was wonderful! I met other pregnant women who were not all French and we were all due one following the next. It turned out that doing yoga was to be something that saved my life yet again. The pregnant women and I ended up becoming close friends, forming a community and stayed in the yoga class all the way until our births. I realized during that time just how valuable and necessary prenatal yoga truly was for me. It was not only to move our pregnant bodies, but for the community building aspect of being together for first time pregnant mothers on the same journey at the same time.

If you have an experienced yoga teacher, it can change not only your life but, also the life inside of you and the destinies of the whole family. I didn't know that with my first son. My prenatal yoga teacher in France had just gotten certified in Hatha yoga, had never been pregnant and she didn't have that much experience with pregnant women doing yoga. Since, she didn't have any experience, she could not help us to feel empowered, nor could she inform or uplift us to have better pregnancies or better births. It was not her fault as she did the best she could in her circumstances and again it was meant to be part of my path in that way. I also realize that I could have been more proactive, too. In any way, looking back I am glad there was a class because I made a life long friend in that class.

Consequently, the experience I had birthing my first son left me with yet another learning experience and it was not at all how I envisioned it to be. I thought I could plan it the way I imagined and not do any other pre-labor work. When the time came, as it was my first birth, I was stuck in the total unknown fear of the experience like a deer in headlights. I had done what I thought was birth preparation classes, I met with a birth preparation emotional support woman with my husband once, but it was not nearly enough of the right method. Therefore, I had not done the work needed to prepare a girl to become a mother and a woman. My birth plan was totally compromised and I was forced to have pitocin and an epidural. This was not how I wanted my baby to come into this world. Plus, it was not my wish to feel completely uncapable, unsupported, uneducated on how to help my baby and myself birth with visualizations and inner dialog. We have a lot of work to do as a society to help women become empowered mothers.

As soon as I arrived at the hospital, I was just another animal or number for the hospital midwives. The same midwives who "prepared" me for my birth day. They were not acting as if they were there because they truly wanted to be helping me. It was just another job for them and they were trying to get through the hours of their shift. The same way that anyone who is not passionate about their job or work can feel during work hours.

My midwife was eating an ice cream in the birthing room and telling me I didn't have enough oxytocin to create contractions, basically she was telling me I was not made to push a baby out of my body. When I finally gave in after being threatened to have a c-section, I took the pitocin in my drip and a half dose of an epidural, but the anesthesiologist was not there. What is worse when she did arrive two hours later, she messed up and had to do two different epidurals into my spinal column. I ended up having my son just fine feeling it all and pushing him out. I pushed him out in like three pushes and I was in total bliss the second he was put onto my chest. The end to that hospital story was magical because I had waited a long time for the beautiful full head of red hair baby boy that I was blessed to hold in my arms after so much waiting.

Despite having done prenatal yoga, I was left with back pain from the epidural for the whole first year of my son's magical life. I loved him more than anything and I was feeling over the moon to have a beautiful baby in my arms, but I felt so unhealthy physically and mentally. I rocked him to sleep every night with pain in my back knowing that it was due to the epidural. I knew that it could have been so different. The back pain mixed with sleep deprivation and a Hashimoto disorder left me feeling half alive, but the Magic of life lifted me inside my mind during that time where my physical body left off. I returned to Hatha yoga after my son was born with the hope that it would help all my "ailments," but it did not.

It was not enough to feel half alive after eighteen months of foggy brain, fatigue, back pain and I was getting depressed, even though I was over the moon to have a baby. I was projecting positivity, support and clear answers during the first years of my son's life and allowing them to come in divine timing. Suddenly my projection about my uncomfortable thyroid issue was answered and the magic re-infused my life. My mom found a new Thyroid doctor and got me new medication that was all natural. The natural thyroid medication helped me begin to feel better and less foggy brained. As my body and mind were being supported through vitamins, natural chiropractors and some acupuncture, I began to see more clearly. My prayers were answered when the Magic decided to move into fifth gear. I remembered some teaching manuals given to me from a friend right before I got married. They were Kundalini yoga teaching manuals and I began doing the yoga at home in small doses. Finally, the energy of total health came to meet my projection of the life I knew was possible.

I remained friends with my prenatal and postnatal French yoga teacher throughout the first year of my baby's life. I went to her with the intention to teach her one Kundalini yoga class and I did! She loved it and told me I had to teach it at her new center. She told me that since she opened her yoga center a couple years prior, she wanted me to teach there. I found myself recharged and inspired to teach this new form of yoga that seemed so different than the Kundalini from fifteen years before. I started teaching with two students and sometimes one student that first summer, but it felt perfectly fit to me. I didn't care whether I had one student or ten because I was developing something huge. After two summer seasons of teaching Kundalini yoga, I had twenty regular students and I loved life on all levels.

It was at that moment another true miracle arrived in my uterus and our lives. I became pregnant without IVF!!! Kundalini had healed us on some level because we conceived naturally. We were surprised, shocked and overjoyed. At the moment when I found out, I made a decision to dedicate myself to a completely conscious birth. I would continue to feel supported by Kundalini yoga and all the gifts it provides when one practices over time. I knew to look for other helpful methods to have the dream birthing experience I was confident would be most magical. I dreamt of the empowered female being I always knew I could be deep down inside to birth the miracle of a baby through me.

I decided to go back to Los Angeles and take prenatal yoga at Golden Bridge Kundalini yoga center in Santa Monica. Once, I did that my birth destiny was fulfilled and my journey was paved. With one step at a time, I rekindled a relationship with Gurmukh and after three prenatal classes and she told me to get her book, "Beautiful, Blissful, Bountiful." From the minute I read her book, my life has been nothing but synchronistic and magical.

To continue to empower my self through the second pregnancy, I sought out learning about hyno-birthing the Mongan Method in France. I continued to teach regular and pre-natal Kundalini yoga and most of my students who came more than five months birthed with no epidural. Decision after decision moved me towards my dream birth experience and my entire pregnancy was healthy. I felt strong, beautiful and empowered and that is what I shared with my students. I taught yoga until a week before I birthed my second son at home, in a birthing pool, while being filmed for a documentary in France.

I have been practicing yoga for 22 years now. As you must have gathered so far, yoga has reminded me how to go deep within myself to the beyond and come back with balance, vitality, and clarity. The truth for me is that I stumbled on the truth that I always hoped would be there; that magic is real. It may sound esoteric or metaphysical, but my yogic journey has led me to discover a reality more real than society's reality.

My first yoga class didn't teach me about this new reality, but it was the first step. The yoga mat has become my magic carpet ride. Every time I step onto it, I discover new things about my inner self and I peel a new layer of awareness. When I am teaching I learn even more. It begins every day when I step onto my mat and I open more; awaken more. What a gift I get to give my self to receive all the beauty and bounty life has to offer and all this from something I never categorized as a career. I am so lucky to have discovered this magical lifestyle of constant self-healing on a deeper and deeper level.

I believe it was not luck, I believe it was my destiny that I kept choosing through the ups and downs. In yogic philosophy, as in Buddhist philosophy, we believe in re-incarnation. What I feel in my current life is that I have already been a yogi in previous lifetimes. I feel that based on various evidences, which I wrote about earlier, but also based on my understanding of Kundalini yoga, life and inner healing. It is as if I remember all of it in some other dimension. I have received clues of information in small parcels regarding yogic philosophy since I was younger, but it was my free will that decided to experiment.

This reminds me of an example from childhood when I received a sign from a movie by Alfonso Cuaron called, "A Little Princess." It is a movie about a young girl, Sarah, who lived in India with her father before WWI and was brought to England during the war while her father went to fight. While living in an all girl's boarding school, she tells mystical stories of living in India. All her stories are historic myths about different Indian gods and goddesses. Many of the Hindu Gods and Goddess stories' had to do with some form of yogic philosophy. Just by looking at depictions of these Gods and Goddesses, we can see if they were enlightened or battling their own emotions such as Goddess Durga; also known as Kali or Paravati. She was the wife of Lord Shiva and the mother of Ganesha, Jyoti and Karttikeya. She was a fierce mother Goddess among the people who fought for peace. She carried many weapons in multiple hands to represent aspects of yogic life such as the conch shell, which represents the sound current when chanting or the trident, which hold many meanings, but one closest to Kundalini is the representation of the three nadi or energy channels in the body the ida, pingala and the central one the Shushmana. Most of the gods and goddesses were striving to be yogis.

Therefore, growing up watching that movie over and over, was a great preparation for me to become a yogi in this life if I wanted to follow the opportunities presented to me. In fact, watching that movie gave me great hope that magic exists; come to find out after discovering Kundalini that not only does magic exist but, it is based in science. Another concept in the movie, also scientifically based was about being able to manifest things before you see them. This concept subliminally mesmerized and taught me how to do it by watching the movie over and over. The princess teaches a girl in servitude, Becky, to dream of having something even though she cannot see it. The two girls imagine a feast and beautiful clothes and in the morning the girls wake up to the very feast they imagined and silk clothes and shoes. The scene was magical in the film and it remains one of the seeds of magic planted in my life all those years ago when my life didn't resemble anything magical at all.

From experiencing all this magic in my life, this is why I believe getting into yoga wherever one is in their lives, can become a tool. Everyone must begin somewhere. Kundalini yoga is meant to be a bonus tool because it creates a practice of focus and grit. Many of my yoga teachers over the years in Hatha or vinyasa would use the anecdote that the body is like a car. If you want to drive your car for a long time, you will make sure to drive slowly, to clean it and to get an oil change every 5000 miles. If you want to drive your body for a long time so that you can enjoy your creations, treat your body as the temple of the soul. That is what Kundalini yoga and meditation is meant to do according to my teacher.

Your body is the vehicle that your soul drives. That is why they call it a temple because your soul is the divine aspect of your physical self. If you can create an idea in your mind, that taking care of your body and your mind by not pushing yourself too hard with work, with play, or with exercise, than your body won't get sick. One step further, in Kundalini yoga we know that if you give your body good fuel, you will stay radiant and young. Yoga is a healing practice that allows one to take care of their body, mind and soul.

Everyone CAN begin to practice yoga with kundalini yoga, but it is not a yoga practice that beginners will immediately enjoy necessarily.

Kundalini yoga and meditation meets us where we are in the moment. It is confrontational because it quickly shows us the limitations in our minds. It would be like asking an agnostic to believe in God and start to go to Church or pray. I did not like it right away because I needed to have more life experience to appreciate the depth and speed of the healing it provides. Some yogis enjoy hard exercise and those types of people already love hatha, vinyasa, ashtanga, Bikram or iyengar styles of yoga, but are not ready to confront their minds. After five to ten years of practicing these other styles, Kundalini yoga and meditation can become more appealing to those types of yogis.

I believe yogic healing is a science and the meditation in Kundalini yoga is what changes the human being from the inside cells out. Those people who do not have any exercise regime can be a good candidate for beginning with Kundalini yoga and meditation because they will not compare it to anything. Finally there are those people that go rogue and use many different styles and forms of exercise or yoga, which work for them. Kundalini yoga and meditation being a cumulative practice that scientifically heals an individual, is a wonderful phenomenon to incorporate into any routine. We all have a childhood and past lives to heal in this lifetime otherwise we face the possibility of karma in the next lifetime.

The beauty of yoga is that, there are millions of ways to practice yoga because it is all yoga. Just as there are millions of people on the planet, there are millions of ways to yoga a life and it looks unique to us all. We are not all supposed to look, act, heal, learn, grow, discover, cry, or die the same way. It is not a competition, it is an acceptance that develops and materializes within over time. The practice teaches us to accept ourselves, just as Gurmukh Kaur Khalsa wrote in her quote I used at the chapter head. She is a monument in the yogic world because of her grace, life experience, perseverance and inner strength to have continued teaching and taking yoga for over forty-five years. As a woman, I am inspired by her to become a graceful human and a teacher like her.

Yogi Bhajan, the master, who brought Kundalini yoga and meditation to the West in secret, said that we must become ten times better than our teachers; meaning him. What he shared is considered ancient wisdom or even the answers to life. He wanted his students to live by these teachings to carry the secret technology to future generations. Of course this is not possible without practicing the yoga and meditation daily, but for me as I have personally seen the magic of it work time and again, I am more than inspired. It is not about touching our toes to our head or standing on our heads that creates the magic to be constantly present in our lives even though it may feel like an accomplishment. It is not about trying to disprove the technology or discredit the teacher either. It is a personal practice to effect our own life. The Kundalini energy can create a space in our minds to see the magic that is already omnipresent. That is why Kundalini yoga must be experienced and not talked about or judged. If we give it a chance for at least six months to a year, our lives can become a magical healing process for humanity.

Kundalini yoga gives an altitude of perspective that is the fastest route to living a magical life. It cuts through all our bull shit. We cannot hang onto our judgements, our limits, our stereotypes, or our past life hang ups, all of which prevent us from becoming magical beings having magical experiences and living in heaven on Earth. If you could be the happiest version of yourself all the time, would you seek out something to ensure that continues or would the change scare you into staying where you are and who you are in this moment? It truly is up to you to decide to continue the cycle of self sabotage or evolve. Try this meditation to make the decision:

Meditation:
To See The Unseen

Sit in easy pose with the spine straight.

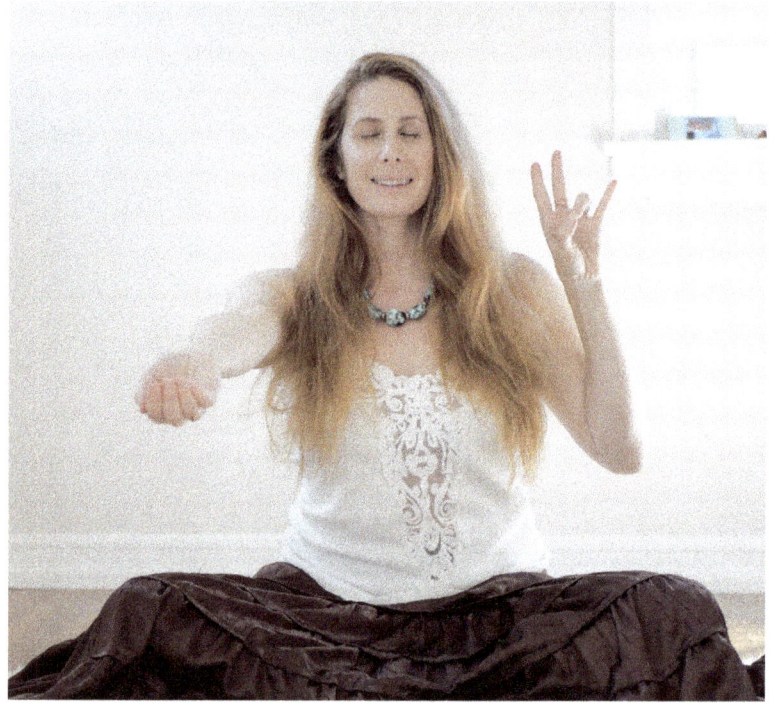

Bend the left elbow near your rib cage while bringing your left hand facing outward. Place your left ring finger (Sun) to touch tip of thumb while all the other fingers point straight up.
Right arm is stretched out in front of you with the right hand cupped.
No bend in right arm.

Close your eyes and focus at the chin. Breathe slowly and deeply consciously listening.

To finish, inhale and maintain for 15-20 seconds as you stretch the right arm forward and squeeze every muscle in your body. Exhale like cannon fire. Repeat 2 times.

Relax for 5 minutes to bring yourself back to normal consciousness. Talk, don't meditate.

This meditation will create for the brain, its' own form of morphine to give the body endurance. Your metabolism will change, the glands will secrete, the nervous system will strengthen and the brain will renew itself.

    If you do this meditation everyday for 120 days with no break and at the same time everyday, it will establish a relationship between your energy and the enhanced energy this meditation provides to your body.

Chapter 5
The Magic of Learning and the Theatre

"Act well your part; there all the honour lies."
    -Alexander Pope

"If you were born with the ability to change someone's perspective or emotions, never waste that gift. It is one of the most powerful gifts God can give-the ability to influence."
    -Shannon L. Alder

"Education is the passport to the future, for tomorrow belongs to those who prepare for it today."
    -Malcolm X

My educational journey was paved similar to many of yours with outer expectations pushed onto us from grandparents, friends, society, and even myself, but I have never been good with pressure from authority. In fact, I tend to run in the other direction because I can feel energy and pushy energy tends to be dark and heavy. (Blessing or curse, feeling energy in extremely empathic ways is called Clairsentience.) If society in America says that we must go to college after high school in order to have a good life, I believe we all must question that society especially when it makes so many mistakes and is void of compassion. This is something I did well as I watched my parents, my teachers and my government fail to have any empathy towards me, my developmental problems based on the many trauma's from my early education or my peers with issues. Which country is getting it right, anyway? It certainly is not America or China, Russia or the EU. We all need to make a global shift of governing together rather than as separate. We are all humans and once, we remember that, things may begin to balance out on Earth.

I was lucky enough to have an English teacher in high school offering a class most seniors wanted to take as an elective. It was titled, Sixties Literature and one day, Mr. Sawajio asked us to think about what we wanted to do after high school and if it included going to college, to sit with that feeling inside. It was a wonderful question to ask us at that time because it made us stop. He was inviting us to go within and not worry about what it looked like from the outside, but it was too little too late for most of us in that class. We were all mostly on the conveyor belt already.

Once we are programmed in our society to go the "normal" route, it is hard to stray and be a pioneer of independent thought. We must be urged from an early age to think independently or else have the inner stamina and self-confidence not to listen to anyone but our self. Most of us as children desire to fit in, to learn early how to conform to our peers in desire of acceptance, but at some point with age we wake up and realize that is impossible. Then we struggle to find our inner voice and our inner drive so that we can discover how to live in this society and world in our own unique way. Our parents were the same and their parents before them; UNTIL NOW. Now, my generation has struggled so much, that more and more, as we become parents are encouraging the new generations of children to be different, to listen to themselves and to break the mold. We are creating a new paradigm because the old one was not working.

My path to this conclusion began to shift after the seed of that sixties literature class was planted because I was already hooked into the belief that college was important for me. I went to an all women's college in Missouri for Theatre and ended up quitting to go to acting school and further ended up graduating from University of California. The shift began slowly to take form as I was presented with decisions about my future. I never knew I could make decisions until my college chapter began to stray from the normal route. My discovery into my educated self began differently and it was thanks to yoga.

At the women's college in Missouri, it was the first time I ever lived for a very long period of time away from family. My mother had a young baby and could not take me to college and so I took myself. I arrived with suitcases in hand and the college counselor who recruited me picked me up. There my experience began at this beautiful 1700's old-fashioned girls school. At first I loved it because we were all in the same experience together, but by the end of the year I had had enough.

I had been studying acting and theatre at Steven's College so upon returning home to Los Angeles, I found an acting school that Jeff Goldblum had opened. It was a wonderful place for a teenager like me trying to understand how to navigate young adult life. I learned more than just acting because of the Sanford Meisner technique of being truthful to the situation I am presented in all moments. This spoke to me on a deep level because I was and had always been seeking the truth. They taught us to be disciplined in our studies and my Tuesday/Thursday class had a great bunch of people.

This lifestyle choice was more my speed compared to college life because I was able to make my own choices while having the protection and comfort of family. I didn't realize all those years ago that I was a clairsentient human, but I had always felt different. I just thought I had issues with emotions. It was when my teacher, Tony Savant at the time, taught a play study class when I began to understand my desire to be an actress. It was a very well written play about Lou Gehrig called, Lou Gehrig Did Not Die Of Cancer, by Jason Miller. The lovely Tony Savant taught it because of its excellent playwriting and also to learn about the importance of a strong spine. I understand today the pure magic as I reflect back to that time from where I am today and how truly every single step I took was to lead me to here. Having a strong, alive and flexible spine in life is part of what I teach through Kundalini yoga.

In studying that theatre piece, we learned how every word, every scene led to more important information in discovering a character. The character of a human is based on how strong or how weak their "spine" is at any moment in their lives and that leads them to make choices about their life on an everyday basis. Therefore, how appropriate that I was learning about playwriting, film writing, and life through studying this one play over a period of several weeks. Excellent education comes in many forms and Tony Savant, Robert Carnegie and Jeff Goldblum have a wonderful program that is Playhouse West/East. It shaped many great people, not all continued to be successful actors like James Franco, Davi Franco, Scott Caan, Ashley Judd and many more, but we all learned so much for our own paths in this life.

My life choices were continuing to shape me into the person I am today forging my own path with a strong, flexible spine and strong self-confidence. After two years of studying with Tony Savant, I moved into Robert Carnegie's class. There, I proceeded to be chiseled by Mr. Carnegie and his magical tough love method. It takes a strong human and a strong teacher to shape and uplift people to their highest potential because it is not easy or fun. Mr. Robert Carnegie is one of those teachers; honest, old school, tough on the outside and all love on the inside.

He saw me through a very important time for a young adult. He watched me, as I vacillated from acting classes to University classes and back to acting classes over a period of six years. He was tough in the best way for young adults who want to work towards a goal. He was leading me towards my education in acting, but on a deep level something inside of me needed healing of a different kind. The kind of healing I probably never received from my childhood and I was stuck on the broken record of my story.

During the time I studied with him, I became better and better at handling my strong emotions, but I still did not comprehend or know of the concept of being a clairsentient at that time. I simply believed I was over sensitive because of my life story and programming from childhood. My ability to feel energy got in the way of my acting abilities because I could feel the energy of my partners and became empathically affected. This threw me off because I was being disrupted in my concentration in our scenes on a subtle level. I did not know that being psychic and deeply empathic was the one ability that made me believe I would be a great actress. I thought since I was very young that because I could feel emotions so deeply, I could absolutely portray those same emotions in acting. I realize all these years later that feeling emotions deeply from others has nothing to do with acting. It has to do with being psychic. Had I known I had this psychic ability and if I could have understood how it worked, perhaps I could have been at ease during the scene.

The tricky thing about being a clairsentient, for me, is that I feel energy and I can read thoughts based on the persons energy. I used to think that other people's thoughts were my own, until I recently in the pas five years I realized I had the ability to read another person's energy even over the phone. Ever since I was young, I was very sensitive to other people's energy and I could not put my finger on why or how it happened. Being so young, so sensitive to other people's energy and so vulnerable in an acting class became too big a challenge for me even older at twenty. After a year and a half, I decided to get some other form of education and life experience by going back to University life at college.

I chose to study Global Studies, which was a new major introduced the year I started. Professors from different departments got together to teach about globalization. I benefitted from having the freedom to design my major from a multitude of subjects relating to socioeconomics, politics, socio-ideological, history and culture. I took the most interesting classes that related to where I was heading and what I wanted to venture into in the future. Again it is wonderfully magical how life truly takes us to where we need to be.

The classes took my mind into the esoteric aspects of globalization and international interests of which I felt a deep desire to learn. I remember many of my professors being wonderful and enthusiastic. Only a handful of classes truly made their mark in my education and for my life. One professor taught my most favorite class, world religions and was also the co-founder of my major. World Religions was my cup of tea because I loved the historical basis from which the information and research was included. Again, this was a complete foreshadow into my future that somehow led me safely towards my destiny. This same professor taught global ethics, which sank in deeply for me as well because the ethics of life goes beyond knowing the Bible; it stems from an intuition that permeates out from every action we create. The philosophical aspects combined with the history from these two classes fulfilled me on a personal level. I felt as if I was learning useful information and I felt compelled to understand.

Global Studies gave me the foundation to a magical protected realm of momentum during that first part of my twenties. I was pushed forward from one thing to the next such as going to France to "perfect my ability to speak French," which led to me wanting to travel to

Thailand, Laos and learning those languages, to meeting multiple people from different cultures and creating a deep compassion for those cultures and beings to deciding upon educating myself through every person I come into contact with as every being has something to teach me for my life. Unbeknownst to me at that early time at UCSB, because when we are young everything looks fragmented, the content I was learning was all connected and leading me to my future life. It was truly the best University experience I could have had.

 All our lives, we are told by society, the media, movies, our friends, our teachers and our parents that going to college can be the most important thing for getting a job and having a good life. More recently, we are starting to see that perhaps it is not this way for every person. Some people need different experiences and are interested in other things that carry them exactly where they want to be. Therefore, a University experience is not pertinent towards having a good life or being happy. We are meant to question what truly makes us happy and if we look at other cultures around the planet, there are happier people who have not gone to University. We are beginning to wake up to the fact that people need to pursue different things to be strong, empowered and happy in their lives. If we could begin to educate our children to their unique specific strengths, then perhaps some kids would grow up knowing better at eighteen if they want to take the time to have a University experience. I am grateful that I chose to finish University because I made the choice for myself and I received what I needed out of that experience.

 Ten years later I went back to Robert Carnegie when I was learning to direct films at New York Film Academy in Hollywood. I still had not discovered Kundalini yoga, but I had written three films and I believed that if I could use my empathic ability to create stories that helped others feel through my directing, I would feel fulfilled. I loved learning to be a director and I had many synchronistic experiences during my time as a student at NYFA. I directed, produced, and edited four short films. It was a great quick education.

Robert Carnegie told me all those years later that I had finally matured. He was proud of me and to see that I was doing something in my potential. To hear those words from him went straight to my heart. He had complimented me and made me feel like I was living within my destiny.

Right upon graduation from NYFA, I returned to France and I booked a producing directing job for my family. They trusted me to create a short film about a new wine they started. Producing it by myself in France where productions are few and far between proved very challenging, but I finished it. Unfortunately, using my cousin as the main character proved to be my one big mistake and my family couldn't use the film for marketing. I followed the script they wanted instead of doing what I had originally proposed. Another big learning experience for me to remember for my future was to always listen to my inner voice.

I learned that directing is hard enough, so, if one is going to produce well, they best hire highly experienced and talented people to work for them. What a great experience for me, but also a clear sign that my destiny was not in directing at that moment in my life. I still have those three screenplays that I wrote almost ten years ago. Perhaps the magic will lead me to a future opportunity to produce those films? I know in my heart that they are stories worth telling to help shift the mindset of society.

I have decided to be a student of life because life is the real teacher and I want to evolve forever. Sometimes we miss the lessons and we need to learn it over and over until we can get above the lesson and integrate it into our lives. It is when we begin to see life as continuous lessons that we can experience our reason for being alive. Life's principles resemble scientific principles because science is true for reality until proven otherwise. Therefore, our lessons in life can be true for us until they evolve. I believe life has so much more to teach me and even that is apart of the Magic.

I am currently studying, among many well-known authors, Ph.D Biologist Dr. Bruce Lipton and Neuroscientist Ph.D Dr. Joe Dispenza for their ongoing studies in their respective fields of study. They are two of the many scientists that are studying the most current ideologies in life, humanity, and our human capacity to self heal, self edudcate, and self evolve. Much of the information being discovered by these two men presently, seems to have been already known by the yogi's of the world in ancient times. My current education is coming to a point where everything is hitting this fever pitch and it is all arriving to the same point or conclusion of origin; as if the information has been surrounding us all our lives, yet hidden in secret.

Dr. Bruce Lipton is well versed in quantum biology and epigenetics and he currently concludes that the mind is the most powerful scientist on the planet. This is what Yogi Bhajan taught for more than forty-five years, while sharing the technology of Kundalini yoga and meditation. He brought the secrets to life here wrapped up in a bow called Kundalini yoga and it is available to anyone who is looking for these answers. Dr. Joe Dispenza gets into how the brain is affected by life and life's challenges after he was in a terrible life threatening accident. He began to heal himself with his thoughts, which led him to look deeper into spontaneous healing; reminding me that even he is on his unique Magical journey of Life to share with the rest of us. Yoga Bhajan says in his teaching and lectures from thousands of years ago that the human is meant to heal itself during our short life journey in the body.

    I am realizing more and more that the Magic is carrying me through my life as if I were on a ride at Disneyland and every turn a new vivid scene full of synchronicity and color unfolds, so that I am able to see one thing completely and become clear for the next. This is how living in the magic of life lifts us to our highest potential as humans one moment to the next. This is also why time is considered by yogis, shamans, priestesses and most awake people to be non-linear. We must not allow ourselves to be programmed by propaganda from the news, television or listening to society telling us how to live our lives because these things do not want you to be awake to your purpose. No one can tell you how to live because YOU came here for a different reason than me. Television is a distraction from life either physically sitting to watch instead of doing something productive or mentally checking out of your busy, stressful life and spiritually it kills the inner feelings of true awareness. Dr. Bruce Lipton says when he is presenting the general feeling of our current civilization that it is bleak unless more of us begin to learn of this new way of being or simply waking up.

    We must be focused on living in the Magic of Life because that gives us energy instead of sucking energy out of us like the television does. It can be easily understood when we compare this idea of having focus on our lives to the image of having focus on a target. If you look away from the target when you let go of the arrow, you will not hit the target. Living in the Magic of Life does not require you to have the same education as I chose. I am sharing these words and this knowledge that I have tediously acquired so that you can allow Life to give you the education you need to understand for your Self. I will end this chapter of education with a funny quote from Yogi Bhajan and the meditation. "You have nine holes, if you control what goes in and out of your nine holes, you will be holy."

Meditation:
Into Being: "I am, I am"

Sit in Easy pose with your chin in jalandhar bandh so the spine is very straight. Your right hand is stretched out and resting on your right knee. Place this hand into gyan mudra (Jupiter tip touches thumb tip.) Your left arm is bent to your left as you place the left hand palm facing your heart.

This meditation has a mantra, the mantra is, "I am, I am." Find the piece of music from Spotify, google or do it without music. It should be slow.

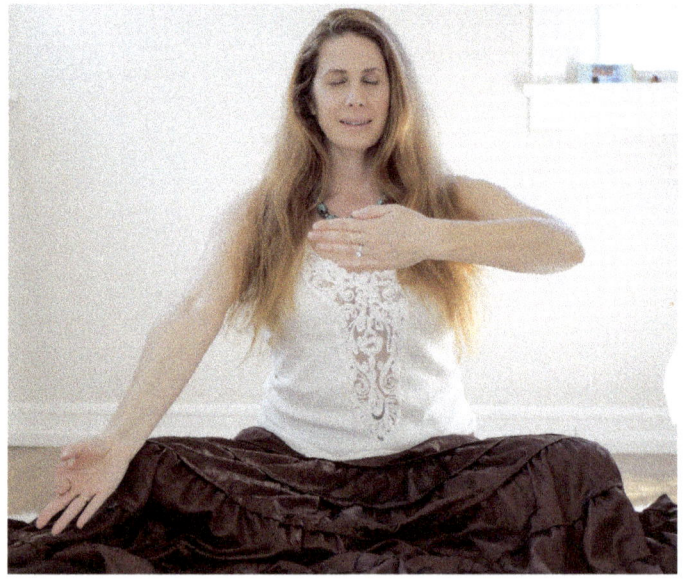

Begin with your left hand 6 inches away from your heart.
As you begin to chant bring your hand closer to your heart 4 inches away.
Then chant the second round as you bring your hand to 12 inches away.

Take a breath in as you bring your left hand back to the first position of 6 inches from the heart.

Continue for 11 min and to end inhale deeply hold and relax completely on your back.

This meditation connects the finite and Infinite identities.

Chapter 6

Drugs, Reiki and Sobriety

"In order to heal we must first forgive...And sometimes the person we must forgive is ourselves."

    -Mila Bron

"Nothing is impossible; the word itself says, 'I'm possible!'"

    -Audrey Hepburn

"I avoid looking forward or backward, and try to keep looking upward."

    -Charlotte Bronte

My hope is that sharing my journey with you, allows you to perceive your own life, like I perceive mine. A meandering road with signs along the side of the road that have always been there to help map out our challenges as we drive through our life and which, have brought you to your present moment. The darker moments are harder to share because of the embarrassment, pain, depression, confusion and disappointment I had to feel to get me to my light and be constantly reborn. Thanks to all the self-help work I have done plus, all the learning through doing and living, I am no longer ashamed to share, to ask for help, or to be transparent about my journey. I understand now that it is much easier on my nervous system and a lot less stressful for my mind to be transparent instead of trying to hide. Furthermore, I believe that if reading my story can help one being get out of their own darkness, just as I got out of my own darkness, than I am meant to help even that one being.

As the paradigm of our world changes, we all can begin to get out of our darkness. In yogic philosophy, as well as in Astrological philosophy it is said that this time is now titled the Aquarian Age. Therefore, it is no mistake that science and technology are catching up to yogic philosophy. The ancient ones or sages have foretold of a time, which is now, where everything will become bright, in the light, and the truth will become apparent. The new science coming out proving this shift into the Aquarian Age is called, quantum mechanics theory. The new mathematics to support this is called fractal geometry. Technology is reaching a point that mimics the power of the human mind, but is nowhere near as powerful as any human mind. In Kundalini yoga, we understand the power of our human mind as being the strongest, fastest super computer to ever exist. Most of us simply do not harness this information unless we're seeking to learn it.

Drugs are definitely a way to find an inner pathway to more experience, but they destroy us at the same time, unless we use them correctly as Shamans are beginning to share or alternative doctors and psychologists. The definition of a drug from Wikipedia is: "any substance (other than food that provides nutritional support) that, when inhaled, injected, smoked, consumed, absorbed via a patch on the skin, dissolved under the tongue causes a physiological change in the body. In pharmacology, a pharmaceutical drug, also called a medication or medicine, is a chemical substance used to treat, cure, prevent, or diagnose a disease or to promote wellbeing. Traditionally drugs were obtained through extraction from medicinal plants, but more recently also by organic synthesis." Re-reading this definition brings up my own experiences with drugs, the experiences I would never partake in now, but also it reminds me of the history of drugs and plant medicine that is so lacking in the definition of drugs.

In ancient times, before science and medicine, there were herbs, plants, berries, trees and nature that were used to heal humans. Now, we are living in a Newtonian world, where we go to see a doctor or pop a pill because humans cannot yet see what could be the matter or the source of the sensation. Instead of being connected from within, we are taught to look outside and to have a person who hardly knows us to identify our ailments. Whether it is a mental ailment, a physical ailment or a spiritual ailment, there is someone who wants us to think that they know better than us. Whereas in ancient times, we had shamans and community medicinal humans who knew us and could describe how to help using what mother earth gave in nature and we would use the group energy to heal our families and friends. Is this such an archaic mentality or can we bring this back in new form?

For me, I was put on an asthma inhaler drug at a very young age, instead of having my community shaman tell my parents that I needed more security within our family dynamic and needless to say, the inhaler did not stop my asthma. The inhaler managed my asthma, but made me feel powerless. I have family members who have been put on albutrin and zanex for their anxiety or mental depression. I know from speaking to them that they also feel powerless, even though the prescribed drug is meant to help or cure them. It took a life or death situation or many life or death situations for me to realize I wanted to cure my asthma, my depression, and my constant negative thoughts. It has taken me a long time to wake up, to become awake, and ultimately to become re-connected to my inner self. This inner Self is the place within me that is becoming my own inner shaman. I am my own medicine woman.

We can all become our own healers and doctors because we all have the most extensive history on ourselves. In fact we are the ONLY ones, but we rely on others for everything, instead of feeling connected and empowered. That is the OPPOSITE to living in the magic of life and it is now the old societal way being proven wrong thanks to an explosion of auto-immune diseases, cancer, thyroid, and many other unexplainable issues that doctors cannot cure. Drugs, just as medicinal plants, herbs and alternative healings have their place in our world, but instead we go outside of ourselves; asking doctors, pastors, parents, and friends.

Instead of turning to our friends, parents, teachers and government we must pick up a book, take a course, listen to a podcast and do some research to learn some insight for our own healing. Dr. Bruce Lipton Ph.D. teaches that it is our belief system, which can purport us into activating our DNA. If we listen to our belief system, we may be able to have cancer or diabetes in our genetics, but not even activate those genes by simply listening to our thoughts. Therefore, we must become open to seeing these dis-eases as an epidemic of the human mind that needs to be attended to on a global level. We need to wake up.

We must begin the conversation with our kids as well, instead of teaching them the old ways of disconnection. If we have children and we care about them, it is our job to create this change. I believe that if we can simply do that, less and less people will turn to drugs for an escape or to self medicate and less people will develop dis-ease. Our society is set up in a way where family is completely disconnected from each other and disconnected from community. It makes sense by the way we progressed as a country to not mimic small tribal villages because we had so much land, but in losing the tribal villages, we lost connection. No inner connection and no outer connection has revealed the damage and flawed way of living on every level; including for Mother Earth.

My drug journey began at thirteen with friends and instead of a spiritual connection or community being available to us, my friends presented me with drugs and alcohol. A friend of mine had an older sibling and she "partied" with other kids her age using their parents' money to buy drugs and alcohol. At that time we were simply looking for more experiences, but using drugs and alcohol to have those experiences instead of something less harmful to our bodies and minds. We were the last generation of kids, which would create an impetus of change.

I smoked my first bong of marijuana at thirteen with the cool older friends. It was the boys who were good looking presenting it in such a way that it was too hard for me to resist. From marijuana, I tried alcohol, ecstasy and mushrooms. My experiences doing drugs were, for me, a way to stretch my mind out in different directions, but I never loved any of the feelings as a way of life. Somewhere deep down, I knew I wasn't addicted like my biological father, but I knew he did drugs and it did not deter me from experimenting. I quickly learned that I was over it on some dimension, but I could never see exactly how to stop completely, when my friends would want to "hang out." It was as if, we were stuck in limiting beliefs about what activities were available.

When I went to college, I continued to attract people who dabbled in drug recreation. At the women's College, I tried opium and continued to smoke marijuana. Then I got into trying cocaine a year later and that still wasn't enough to get me past the hump of realizing that drugs were never going to be a way to have a higher life experience. It wasn't until I went to Thailand that my life gave me an experience beyond control.

I went to Thailand for six months as a life changing experience that my boyfriend at the time described to me as something amazing to do. I was already interested in traveling because as I explained earlier, I love having that type of experience shape my character and personality. This trip was the most pivotal moment of my entire life because it wrapped all my fears, insecurities, low self-confidence and immaturity together in one big wave of a wake up call. My boyfriend at the time smoked more marijuana than I had ever seen before and I made a decision that if I was to be with him, I had to do the same thing. We smoked joints from what felt like morning until night, but I was doing it against my true intuition.

When we got to Thailand, we smoked from Thai bongs from what felt like morning until night. We were functional drug addicts. Then after three months of living in Thailand and Laos, we were meant to celebrate the New Year. The night of New Year's Eve 2001 I thought getting Thai "ecstacy" would be a really amazing and memorable New Year's Eve. It turned out that the "Thai ecstacy" was actually a drug called, "Yabba" and it was killing Thai people all over Thailand. Our wonderful New Year's Eve turned into a week-long nightmare for me that I could not stop.

I got stuck in the mind's deficiency to quickly release the drug out of my body from whatever chemical was in the Yabba. All my fears, insecurities, and low self-confidence were taking over my ability to think clearly. In fact, reality was even becoming different and bizarre to a point that I was seeing different dimensions and what I thought to be different time periods. I saw images of being alive in Egypt with the pyramids and having memories from what happened to me during that time. I remember this as if it were yesterday because I was truly living that nightmare and felt so stuck; which, is exactly what neuroscientists have recently proved for what the mind is capable of doing. Moreover, it is what we are all doing every day. We believe our mind and the illusion of a world the mind creates and then live in that world. If one can visualize something in their own mind, such as winning the

Olympics, it can then repeat itself in reality with sufficient training and repetition, which is what some master coaches teach their athletes to do.

The five days it took for the Yabba to get out of my body were the most terrifying and scary days of my life. I called my mom around the fifth day and told her what was going on from my point of view. I told her my boyfriend was trying to kill me and many other horrible and crazy scenarios. Luckily she sobered me up immediately. She said, "you are on a cliff created by your thoughts and either you fall off the cliff and live in this mind frame for the rest of your life, or you take steps to snap out of it." It was something only a mother, my mother, could do being in Thailand from where she was in Southern California and it worked.

I got out of Thailand with my boyfriend and a few weeks later I was in Southern California. I was back at my parents' house sobering up and that is when things really began to get interesting on my journey into real magical living. I began eating vegan and then raw because I happened to get a job working for a raw restaurant owned by a celebrity chef named, Juliano's Raw. He began teaching me how to eat raw and cook food with a dehydrator. The food was actually very tasty and I was feeling so clean and healthy. I began exercising for three hours a day and that was my daily routine for two months straight.

My mental state was healing and coming back to reality slowly with every new day because I was reading self help books such as, "Anatomy of the Spirit" by Caroline Myss, "The Four Agreements" by Don Miguel Ruiz, "The Alchemist" by Paulo Coelho, "Same Soul, Many Bodies" by Brian Weiss, writings by Marianne Williamson and "You Can Heal Your Life" by Louise L. Hay to name a few I remember. These books led to my first step in healing my temporary out of mind experience from the disastrous choice I made in Thailand to take drugs. That was 2002 and that was the last time I ever did any drugs.

To further help me heal my mind, I was introduced to a friend of my mothers who happened to be a Reiki Healer. Coincidently, but not, her name was the same as my mother's. Diana knew my mother from twenty years before when she was one of my mothers' birth doula for her underwater birth. Diana helped my mom labor my younger sister into this world in one of the first underwater births. They had lost touch over the years, but my mom still had Diana's number and this time the need was dire because my mental health was at risk.

Diana lived on Abbot Kinney Avenue in Venice with her husband who owned an antique shop. She practiced Reiki healing, crystal healing therapy and guided meditation. In 2002, Abbot Kinney Ave. was still in the transition phase from small eclectic businesses and cute old Venice houses to the modern revamped millennial playground it is now. Diana's healing studio was upstairs from the main house that held all sorts of antique collectibles sold by her husband. The whole house felt like a different world holding open a vortex of powerful energy upon leaving the street behind. Walking through those doors was already attention grabbing.

This experience was another part of my journey towards destiny because I was being pushed forward from an invisible power in synchronistic manner. Looking back in retrospect, I realize yet again how true having a strong belief in our innate ability to find our personal destiny must be. The Magic was what was pulling me into limitless and conscious living. That first visit with Diana, she explained to me what she did as being a mix of Reiki and healing. She was so nurturing and calm that I immediately felt taken care of, protected and safe. This first healing visit, my mom came in the room with me. While I lay on a massage table Diana began by talking with an extremely strong yet, warm voice and by placing her hands above my closed eyes.

    She began speaking introductory phrases that she intuitively picked up on with the smallest amount of background history such as, "it is not your fault," "you're innocent," and "you are safe here to know that your mother loves you and she always has and always will." I remember having thoughts of distrust, rejection, betrayal, and low self-esteem, from my childhood all the way until Thailand bubbling up in my mind as listened to her voice. While this mental process occurred a physical exemplification of release simultaneously began as I was crying and crying and crying. While she continued placing her warm hands above my heart, then down my body hovering over it as if checking for stagnant energy or heat, I felt bathed in the warmest protective light of my whole life. Whatever she was doing was so very therapeutic and her voice was so soothing that I could have fallen asleep into bliss.

    Following the session, Diana led me to her upstairs living room/kitchen where there were stones and crystals everywhere. She sat me down in a chair with a drawing underneath the chair over the floor in the middle of the room. She began to explain to me what Reiki was and how she practiced it. She explained how Reiki was an energetic type of healing that is done through the hands and anyone can utilize this modality. She initiated me to be a Reiki practitioner at that moment if I ever had a desire to heal others. Finally she asked me to go pick out any stone in the room.

I chose a triangular burnt orange jasper stone that was easy to hold between two fingers. She led me to hold this stone while speaking affirmations into it. She said that I should say a new affirmation everyday all day into the stone. Then the next day change the affirmation. She wrote down many affirmations for me on 3x5 cards. She said to rub the stone as part of a meditation for self-healing, while repeating the affirmations. She also gave me a mantra to speak in Sanskrit.

I did everything Diana told me to do and I continued to get treated by her over a period of three months. She was helping me to see the light positive side of life and teaching me to energetically lift my own vibration. It all sounds funny now writing about it, but during this process, I felt like she was saving me. It sounds almost like a hoax to some people to do this type of healing work. The Church said that witches of the ancient times were devil worshiping when practicing these types of rituals to dissuade the society from belief, but in the Pagan wisdom this was the way to heal. All the therapies, rituals, traditions and beliefs from that ancient time now feels more real to me than ever. The last session I had with her was one of the most amazing and unexplainable experiences total. I am still to this day unsure if it was real or something she did.

I walked in like I did every other time to see Diana for my session, but this time I found her in the back of the antique shop and not upstairs. She explained to me that this final treatment would be down stairs in one of the rooms in the back of the antique store because her and her husband had decided to sell the house. Therefore, they were using the whole upstairs portion for packing. She directed me to the room where our session would be and I realized this house/antique store was a real mystery that kept inventing new rooms I had never seen before; almost like a carnival fun house perfectly aligned with the enigma of what had occurred with me throughout that three month period of healing. I lain down on the massage table and she began checking my energy with her hands and speaking to me in her same relaxing, calming manner.

    I began relaxing and listening to her talk about my vibration and light filled energy. I got into such a relaxed state that I was either in a deep meditation, asleep or almost asleep. All of a sudden, I felt I was alone. Diana had left the room for me to relax on my own and I could hear what seemed to be angels singing or humming. It sounded like thousands of voices at the most perfect, angelic pitch all singing at once into my ears. The music became louder and louder, but never deafeningly loud. I opened my eyes and looked around, but while Diana had returned, she wasn't singing. The music continued and I just listened to the sound of what I can only describe as a heavenly choir of angels. It began to slowly fade away and she soon interrupted to explain that she was finished with my session. I sat up and immediately asked Diana if she heard any music. She only responded, "no." How could that be possible??????? I still to this day am in the mystery of that sound. With all the research I have done on the internet, I have never found or heard anything like it since.

    Succeeding in my life past that lost place at thirteen tasting pot for the first time and feeling unsupported by my friends and family through to age twenty-four upon taking an illegal drug in another country until now, I truly realize that our society needs a new narrative regarding drugs, healing and medicine. Thirteen is simply too young to experiment with any kind of drug; let alone become addicted. Perhaps if our government, police, parents, teachers, doctors and friends could see drug use as a call for help, our whole world would change. This new paradigm is igniting massive change on every level of our lives because we are waking up to creating real solutions to previously unresolved problems. The Universe is here to help push us forward in our evolution.

We are not turning to churches for all our answers. We are not turning to doctors to heal us because they are working with the pharmaceutical companies who are killing us. We are not turning to onetime scientific theories, which spoke about life being a survival of the fittest. The newest science is catching up with the oldest most ancient yogic philosophy and so must we individually. Yogi Bhajan and Bruce Lipton both say that we must become our own doctors, our own chefs and our own healers.

Simply put, when we feel our life puts us in between a rock and a hard place, that is the exact moment we need to focus our senses on shifting to spaciousness within. If we cannot create that within our body, mind or energetic field on our own, we must seek outside help with homeopathic remedies, energetic healing, astrological reading, Akashic record reading, or simple old tarot cards and that can make the first shift for us. These outer reinforcements are not meant to make us feel shameful, guilty or powerless in any form. They are simply a higher guidance system sending in extra help.

The following meditation is literally titled, Medical Meditation For Mental Habituation. If we are to turn to ourselves to fix our physical dis-eases, mental dis-eases and addictions, whether be it negative thinking, chocolate, drugs, alcohol, smoking, or un-happy relationships, the following meditation is the medicine and the work to heal. We all have occasional times of treating our bodies in toxic manners and having toxic beliefs that remain in our lives, but are no longer true. To rid ourself of these addictive patterns and beliefs becomes a mind battle, but this meditation will make it easier and doable. How badly do you want to create new patterns, be healthier, be gentler to yourself, and manifest true happiness in your daily life and life perspective?

Medical Meditation
For
Mental Habituation

To begin sit in easy pose and bring your fingertips curled into the palm so that every fingertip touches the padding in the palm.

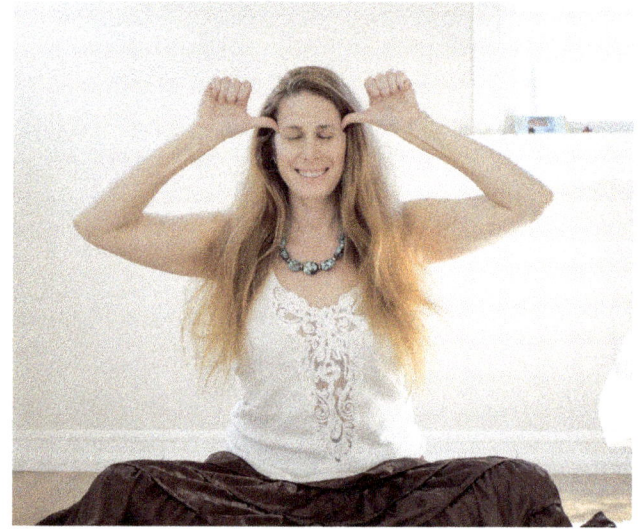

Place the thumbs to your temples on each side.
Gently push onto the temples as you squeeze the back molars together.

As you squeeze the molars together, begin mentally saying, "Sa, Ta, Na, Ma" rhythmically; one word per squeeze.

Focus your eyes up to the third eye or brow point.
Repeat the sequence for 5 minutes to begin.
Then slowly work to 31 minutes.

Do it for 40 days to break an addiction or habit.

Chapter 7
Cannes Film Festival =Magic

"I think cinema, movies, and magic have always been closely associated. The very earliest people who made film were magicians."
    -Francis Ford Coppola

"Even though I make those movies, I find myself wishing that more of those magic moments could happen in real life."
    -Jane Seymour

"I've been to Cannes 15 or 16 times, and every time I go, there's a kind of soul-stirring feeling."
    -Gong L

After months of seeing Diana, I truly did feel better physically and stronger emotionally, mentally and energetically. I suppose at that time, I did feel my "vibration" was becoming higher. She was teaching me for over two months that in life like attracts like. I began to believe it, even without understanding it completely I was doing the work of believing before seeing. I could feel something on a deeper level brewing from all this high vibration work. I finally convinced myself of my ability to manifest miracles even when the outer world showed no proof. I continued to believe in what Diana taught me and in the following few weeks, a poignant proof to her teachings manifested into an experience beyond my wildest dreams. It was pure magic.

I will set you up with the entire story leading up to this most magical manifestation. Reiterating on a linear timeline that the previous year I finished college at UCSB and because I had wanted to become an actress even before UCSB, that feeling of working in film came back after I healed from my out of mind experience in Thailand. I graduated in March of 2001 and immediately I got a job assisting a film production company in Pacific Palisades, California. They hired me because my mom was close to them, but also thanks to my background with French and France. The CEO's decided when they hired me to go to the Cannes Film Festival and they would pay for me to work as their assistant at the festival.

I decided to work at the film festival that year and then stay my second summer in France. I would live with my boyfriend and work at the beach clubs again like the year before. I learned the lay of the land at the Cannes film festival as the assistant to the CEO's. I walked along La Croisette hundreds of times, I checked out films to see which would be interesting to possibly buy for distribution, I prepared all the meetings and took minutes for some and I was able to enjoy the generosity of my bosses. Because Cannes during the Film Festival is a whole huge production of its own, it was important that first year attending to see how to work the film festival side of the production.

Following the film festival, my bosses left a few days before the last day when all the films get picked for prizes. We went to St. Tropez to show my bosses where my family lived and discuss certain decisions my bosses were thinking of making during the festival. Then, they left me with my boyfriend and I continued with my plan to stay the summer. With so much free time on my hands, I went to the beautiful beaches on the Mediterranean Sea a lot. Most of the time, I would go to the beach where my boyfriend worked.

The day after the festival ended, there was a big table at the beach club and everyone was French except for one American man. I already knew some people at the table and I was invited to join them for lunch. As I was talking about my experience during the film festival, the American overheard me talking and began to tell me about his production company, based in Santa Monica. I told him that I was born and raised in Santa Monica and he invited me to give him a call the following year if I wanted "to truly learn about the Cannes Film Festival and Film Market." I had kept his offer in the back of my mind and proceeded to have a wonderful summer. The following Fall and Winter was for my trip to Thailand.

Fast forward to post Thailand and my three-month energy healing to raise my vibration with Diana. Feeling so good after a month of treatments, I made a decision not to live in my fearful thoughts, which prevented me from doing anything too scary. Remembering the offer from that man back in Saint Tropez the year before, I thought perhaps I could get a job with him. I decided to give him a call to test my progress after a month.

At that time, Marshall Heuser told me over the phone that he had an assistant at that time and wasn't sure if he would need another assistant in Cannes that year. I thanked him and let it go for the Universe to take over, as I was practicing the principles of raising my vibration Diana had taught me; all the while feeling very confident that something good would happen. Two months went by and then I received the call five days before Cannes was to start. Mr. Heuser over the phone says, "if you still want to go to Cannes you have to leave in three days." He told me that I would go in advance on a flight through London then to Cannes and prepare the office in the hotel, get our badges and begin setting up meetings. When I asked my mom what she thought, she said absolutely not because I did not know him well and I needed to think logically. I was too busy bouncing off the walls with excitement and I responded "yes" that night to this man I did not know well.

There I was, three days later getting packed to go back yet again to Cannes. This time it was for a very inspiring reason; my dreams and my vibrations. I had always wanted to work creatively in the film industry whether as an actress, writer, producer, or director. Here I was thinking this is my chance to make it happen. I was clear headed, determined and filled with lighter vibrations. The day came when I was to leave and it was also Mother's Day. My flight was scheduled at 11:15 p.m. so I got to spend the day with my mom and my family, then leave on my dreamy adventure.

The British Airways flight pulls into the sky and I can see the evening lights of Los Angeles below me. The glow seems to be cheering me on for this adventure as if it were the magical opportunity that would change my life forever. I am so excited with all these ideas swirling around inside my head that I don't even sleep. I simply converse with a scientist from Indonesia who imports coconuts to Germany where they make oil. He was so interesting that I didn't even see the time pass. We talked almost the whole flight. The next thing I know the plane is landing and this nice man convinces me to go out into London during my five-hour layover. He hands me 50 pounds sterling and says, "Have a wonderful trip in Cannes!"

Synchronicities continued the moment I stepped off the plane and said thank you to the nice man and out into the Heathrow terminal. I met a girl named Hannah walking off the plane who also wanted to go into London during her layover. We took the Heathrow express to Paddington Station and got off just as the Indonesian man explained to me. She and I walked out into London and it was as if I was in a film already.

We saw a beautiful big green park to our left and the double deck red bus of London to our right. Everywhere was so clean and royal. It was my first time in London and I filled my senses up with as much as I could in that short layover. Hannah and I looked around at shops and we found a quaint little café for a quick coffee in Oxford Square. As soon as we stepped into the café, it began to rain. Queue the rain, the wind, and the total package of romantic London weather for us as a backdrop to our break in the cafe.

The man who served us our coffee was French, named Regis and happened to be from Cannes. That moment it seemed the Universe was playing a joke on me, winking at me and putting me into a beautiful twilight zone of goodness. My boss from the beach club restaurant who took my boyfriend and I to Thailand was also named Regis. I explained to coffee shop Regis that I was on my way to Cannes for the Film Festival and I began to think to myself how perfect that day was unfolding. It stopped raining and Hannah and I decided to go explore a little more. So, I paid for our coffees with the money the Indonesian man had given me and we went to a park and then bought some gifts for her family.

Back at Heathrow Airport, I say goodbye to Hannah as she leaves for Germany and I made my way to the British Airways executive lounge. I pass the sliding doors and see two women welcoming travelers and asking for their membership cards. Instead of stopping, I simply walk right past them as if I belonged and they did not stop me. It was another miracle. I ended up staying in the lounge for an hour to relax and enjoyed finger sandwiches, tea, cookies, newspapers, magazines, a shower and T.V.

I arrived in Cannes and jumped into a taxi at the airport. The taxi drops me off in front of the Carlton Hotel in the center of La Croisette in Cannes. Walking up to the front door, I felt like royalty with the hugest smile on my face. It mattered not that I was an assistant to a producer, I felt like I had arrived to the top of my game elevated to royalty in front of everyone. The doorman took my suitcases and I began to literally pinch myself. I walked to the front desk and announced my name. The bellman directed me to the rooms where we would be staying for two weeks. When he opens the door to my room, the exhilaration takes over my whole entire body. My room over looked the Mediterranean Sea and La Croisette. My room is so beautiful with the most beautiful bed, desk, and the most beautiful bathroom I had ever seen. The bellman left me and I began jumping on the bed with such an overwhelming excitement. I was able to look out over the Mediterranean Sea mid jumps to see the lights from the preparation of the festival. My vibration was unquestionably heavenly.

That first night I could not even sleep, I was so excited. In the middle of the night I found myself in the most gorgeous room in the world doing yoga. I discerned that making the decision to come was the best thing I would ever do and the reward was already huge. The next morning croissants, pain au chocolats, and coffee were brought to my room. I grasped at that moment that this trip was simply getting better and better. I unpacked my clothes and set the office up.

Feeling grateful I worked the year before in Cannes, I already knew where everything was situated. So, I took care of registration. At registration, I met a wonderful girl who tells me how she was on my flight from London and she noticed me. We ended up grabbing lunch and she finishes helping me set up the festival office in my hotel room. My boss arrived that afternoon and he took me out to dinner to discuss his schedule for the following two weeks that I was to be his assistant. I became conscious in that moment of the fact that my Reiki treatments truly worked because no matter what I was doing for my boss or how mundane, it was exciting to me and I kept my vibration high by repeating my mantra and affirmations.

It was as if I was seeing life with new eyes, like in the movie Limitless, where Bradley Cooper takes the drug and he can see the matrix of the world. I would go shopping for him and meet people everywhere I went. While I went out to drop off or pick up his dry cleaning, I saw movie stars or I got free coffee from different cafés. I was feeling like the star of my own movie and then the festival began. That evening was like the opening of a concert when the singer first comes onstage. I felt this rush of Euphoria come over me from what I would see and experience during my time in those two weeks. My boss took me to every event as he had invitations to mostly all of the parties. He taught me all about the industry at that time and he even let me sell the rights to Romania and Thailand for a film he was pre-selling.

The two weeks were flying by and I was sleeping 4 hours or less a night due to sheer excitement. On the fourth night after two nights of yacht parties, rooftop of hotel fashion shows, and beach club dinners we went to Hotel Martinez down the street for a drink. He ended up introducing me to a group of producers who were the young power players for that year. They were the ones doing all the deals with the big studios and larger production companies. They were seemingly nice and we became one big group going around together every night after the deals were made. They invited me to amazing parties and movie screenings. The next day they picked me up in a Mercedes limousine and they invited me to Jay-Z's house party at the most amazing mansion I have ever seen in Antibes.

The next night a group of us went out to a club and they wouldn't let the guys in because they were not wearing tuxedos, but when I went up to the door man to work my magic, I looked into his eyes, spoke

French and then he let us all in, but not before he looked straight into my eyes and said in French, "la plus belle, celle-la." I began to feel like I could do or manifest anything I could imagine. Inside all the parties we saw movie star after movie star and received gift bag after gift bag while dancing the night away. Every night was bigger and better than the one before. Every day was full of me being successful on every level and I thought to myself, "I never want this moment to end."

    I realized that I was staying connected to my inner self and it felt so good and I felt so powerful and so uplifted. It was palpable how magical my reality was yet, how unexplainable it could sound to anyone else. I began to ask myself to manifest something even more amazing to test my ability to co-create with whatever it was that was controlling all this manifesting. The next day, I was working in the office and a guy came in to talk to my boss. He begins telling me that he has no one to go with to the famous Amfar Aids event that Elton John puts on every year in the following days. I told him that I would love to go with him, but that I did not have anything to wear.

    The next day he brought me to a boutique to buy me a new dress and shoes!!! It was miraculous-ness in motion because literally all I had to do was think about something I wanted, without being attached to the result and it would happen even better than my imagination. That night I went out with the guys, who were becoming like brothers, as I had been doing every night. This time they brought me to the Noga Hilton dance club VIP room and since I love to dance, I got up on one of the speakers. I was wearing flipflops with a fun outfit I had bought in Thailand and I just let go. As I was dancing on that speaker, a new guy, Matthew had come out with us all that night and he came up to me and literally asked me what I wanted to do with my life. He told me if someone could look that amazing dancing on top of a speaker wearing flipflops, he wanted to help me achieve whatever I wanted. That was the best pick up line I had ever heard.

Later that night we went to a house party and met some famous soccer players and a famous designer named Von Dutch who was literally cutting t-shirts that girls were wearing on their bodies. He was at this rented house in the kitchen cutting new styles. I spent the entire night with Matthew and on some level I was falling in love with him. I had not had any alcohol or drugs the whole time because I was already so high on my own inner power. Matt told me that he also was sober.

When we left at four in the morning, everyone wanted to go out to another party, but Matthew and I went back to my hotel room/ office and took a bath together in our bathing suits. He explained that he was a producer and how hard he had to work to get where he wanted to go. We talked about our lives and I felt like he was a real gentleman. I felt like Julia Roberts in Pretty Woman and he was my Richard Gere. We talked and talked and talked as if time was standing still. We were in different dimension of connection than I have ever felt. We laughed and made inside jokes like we were creating a lifetime in that one morning. We spent the rest of the morning together in the bath.

At seven thirty a.m. he walked me out to get my bosses dry cleaning and he asked me what I wanted to be again. He said that he could make me into a movie star. He was saying the exact words I wanted to hear, but it must have struck a chord in my subconscious programming because I hesitated. I began to feel the first pang of inner self-doubt since my healing with Diana. My fears started to take over the end of that conversation because I responded, "I will let you know when I am ready." He then asked me to go with him on a trip to Germany the next night for a meeting, but I couldn't get out of the fear. I wanted to go with him so badly because I was falling in love with him, but I had planned to go to Amfar and finish my job with the producer. So, I let him slip out of my hands.

That night was the Aids Gala, AMFAR and I didn't want to miss it. I worked all day and my boss let me stop early to get ready. It began to rain late in the afternoon as I was getting ready. I went downstairs to the lobby to wait for the man to pick me up and just when he arrived, I began to pray that it would stop raining long enough for me to not get my hair wet. Literally the minute I put my foot outside to get into the limousine, it stopped raining. I thought to myself, "WHAT now I can control the weather?!?!"

When we arrived in Mougins, which was located on the mountain above Cannes, there was a red carpet and a photographer friend that I had met on the plane from London who was there as a paparazzi. He snapped some photos of me on the red carpet and I felt like a movie star. When we got into the restaurant, a silent auction was taking place at the same time as an aperatif. We ate some hors d'ouvres and browsed the auction area. There were trips, jewelry, tennis lessons with André Agassi, boats, etc. I found a trip to Italy and I immediately wanted to bid on it and go there with Matthew, but I realized that I missed that opportunity just at that moment and I had a deep pang of sadness knowing I was dreaming.

Right when I began to get sad, my date grabbed my arm and led me to the garden. There, we met David Lynch, his wife, Adrian Brody and his parents. This beautiful night was just getting started and it was something that I had manifested for myself. So, I thought I needed to be feeling grateful instead of sad and I immediately shifted my energy. The dinner began and we were ushered into a huge tent with tables decorated as if for a wedding. In the back of the tent a wall of paparazzi were shooting photos of all the famous faces sitting at the tables next to ours. Sharon Stone walked out to begin a presentation of the live auction. A friend of my dates bought a huge diamond necklace for his wife right off of Sharon Stone's neck. He was sitting at our table, which was centered right in front of the stage, and Sharon came and sat on his lap to give him the necklace. Sharon is truly one super sales girl. She continued to sell tennis lessons to Prince Albert for 100,000 dollars that night and some other things.

The night continued with Elton John performing, "That's why they call it the blues" among others. Milla Jovovich sang with Sharon Stone on stage and they asked a bunch of girls to come up on stage to dance with them. Of course I was one of them because it does not take much to get me to dance. Next, Harvey Weinstein got on stage to present the next performer and realized he had a couple of minutes that were unplanned. He asked the audience "if there was anyone who wanted to get a meeting with him for a couple of minutes now was the time." Inside my body I wanted to jump out of my chair and onto that stage to talk to him. This guy, Harrison, who was also one of the guys becoming like a brother to me was at my table and he looked at me as if to say get up there. Something in that moment stopped me from jumping up to tell Harvey Weinstein that I was meant to be a movie star and I have been kicking myself in the mind ever since. I thought that I missed another opportunity right in front of my face due to fear.

I have regretted those two missed opportunities for over ten years and I've often asked myself why I couldn't simply say yes. Moreover, I have contacted and re-contacted those two men to try and ignite a new opportunity, but the moment had passed and we cannot ever go back. I realize that decisions made out of fear, those that hold us back from jumping, will change the course of our destiny forever. Although if we eventually make the course correction to heal fear, our destiny can turn out better than that original possibility. As it turns out all these years later that perhaps I was protected by my fear or my angels in those instances by now seeing how abusive Mr. Weinstein treated women. What I can reflect upon from those missed opportunities is that, we can never be totally without fear, but when opportunities fall in front of your lap, say yes anyway. We cannot let fear limit us because all fear is, is a test.

The AMFAR evening was nonetheless beyond magical. It simply solidifies my belief that every instance in our life shapes our destiny, including the missed opportunities. It truly becomes a question of whether we learn from them or not. I don't regret my decisions anymore because I know that I am constantly raising my vibration everyday now. This time, I have wisdom to persevere through the challenges and the fear. Through this book, teaching Kundalini yoga and meditation, having a podcast, giving motivational talks, holding workshops and private healing with goal clarification sessions all over the world and creating products, I am living with a higher vibration all the time to attract magical opportunities into my life. Plus, I get to serve humanity by sharing to help others live their destiny. This is the true gift because in my heart I believe it is this that can help the Earth raise its' vibration.

Cannes ended beautifully, magically and it remains the most exciting two weeks of my past. The last day of the festival my boss took me to the Carlton Hotel beach buffet for one last lunch meeting. It was a moment of perfection to be imprinted into my cells memory forever. Despite the sadness of it being the end of my adventure in Cannes, I was still over the moon from the experience. I got on the British Airways flight to London with a smile from ear to ear. Of course when I got to London, I went back to the executive lounge to relax and to write in my journal about everything that had happened in Cannes. I wrote down every person I met, every experience I lived so that I would never forget. Who knew all these years later, I would put that experience into a book. When we are living in love, instead of fear or hate, our whole experience of life becomes magical. I can say this because I've lived it and it remains my core belief.

Meditation:
Solve Communication Problems

This meditation activates the Mercury power, which is the power of communication. It clears the ability to perceive all the best ways to speak from other useless chatter. It can create opportunities through high frequency speech; bringing the polarity of all your seeds planted by the words you speak.

Sit in easy pose and bring the hands facing the ground 3 to 4 inches in front of the center of the chest.

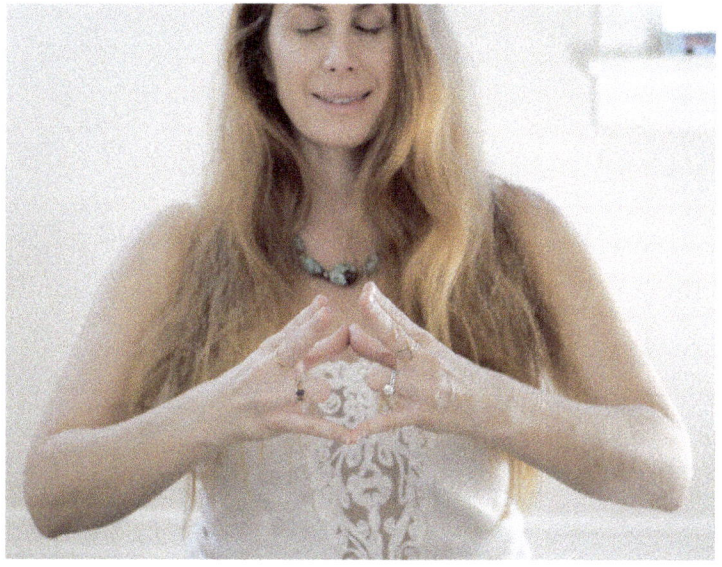

Touch the thumb and Mercury finger of one hand to the thumb and Mercury finger of the other hand. Bend the sun (ring) fingers down towards the palm. Both sun fingers do not touch the palms. Leave the Jupiter and Saturn fingers straight up and not together.

As seen in the photo, leave the hands in this mudra to meditate while listening to "Beloved God" song of Snatum Kaur's.

11 min.

Simply sit breathing as slowly as you can with your eyes closed looking up at your brow point and really listen.

Chapter 8

Spirituality

"Ego says, 'Once everything falls into place, I'll feel peace.' Spirit says, 'Find your peace, and then everything will fall into place.'"

    -Marianne Williamson

"I belong to no religion. My religion is love. Every heart is my temple"

    -Rumi

"Make your own Bible…"

    -Ralph Waldo Emerson

"We are not human beings having a spiritual experience. We are spiritual beings having a human experience."

    -Pierre Teilhard de Chardin

I have a belief in my mind that says, "religion and Spirituality are not the same." Although they are often thought of as one, the differences for me between organized religion and Spirituality are like night and day, quite literally. And for me Spirituality pre-dates religion and it will last throughout all of time well into the future. Religion is also dogmatic and Spirituality is about light and high vibration. As science advances through the leaps discovered in quantum mechanics, quantum physics, Biology, Neuroplasticity and technology it pushes the stagnant places in our society, such as religion and medicine forward at light speed, shifting the construct of our society into the new paradigm of thinking and believing.

This new paradigm is hinting towards whole new ways of seeing our world and therefore, like a domino affect the construction of government, community, society, education and our whole perspective on lifestyle needs to change. Thanks to meditation I already have begun to shift into the new paradigm in my own life. I suppose in a good way my life has set me up to be one of the pioneers of the shift for the good of humanity by everything I speak about in this book. I will be steady, ready for the shift and welcoming the Age of Aquarius with open arms. Dr. Bruce Lipton Ph.D says that this current stage of reality is shifting because of three questions humanity asks and to whom we look to for our answers.

I like the way he designs this perspective shift simply, because it is congruent to ancient yogic philosophy as far as I have discovered. His three questions are, "Who are we? Where do we come from? What do we do while we are here?" He reminds us that in history at some point humanity answered these three questions from the perspective of the native peoples. Then, as time continued, we were manipulated to look to the Church and the people inside the churches, synagogues, mosques, etc. for our three responses. It was a different paradigm and one that the creator created where in order for all of humanity to grow stronger we had to pass through the darkness of religion. We have all heard the stories of what priests did to boys in the Catholic tradition, or how most Pastors and Rabbis counsel their parish and aggregation to listen to only them, or finally how we have to give away our money and worldly possessions to the Church and be accepted by God.

Now is the paradigm where science, mystics, yogis, native peoples and the rest of humanity are beginning to remember a different set of responses to the three questions Dr. Bruce Lipton Ph.D. spoke about. The sages and ancient ones have foretold of a time when people were going to begin to find the answers they are seeking inside of themselves. For me, I believe that the ancient sages knew that if they gave the secrets too early in our evolution, we would have destroyed all of it. We as a young race of humans needed to work to get past the ignorance and darkness so that all of us could make the shift together for the planet and the multiverses outside of our Milky Way galaxy. Perhaps one planet at a time is now waking up to create a new Magic for all Creation.

In the science of quantum mechanics, scientists are discovering and proving what we are truly made of at the center of our cells. They have discovered that matter is not what we have all been told to believe it is; which is dense, heavy and dead. They are discovering that matter is in fact energy and WE are also energy at our core nucleus. The ancient sages spoke of our human bodies as beings of light and vibration, hence the universal language of music; vibrations make sound. Truly at our core, we are "spinning energy vortices with light photons bouncing off to create the illusion of a body or a couch, chair or wall" explains Dr. Bruce Lipton Ph.D.

Upon learning this, I believe our whole paradigm is shifting because that old belief that someone has to tell you how to be or how to heal or how to live is now over. Therefore, it is no surprise that the time for religion is ending as well. Organized religion served its purpose in creating a way of organizing community, but instead of using the truth once the community was created, they used lies and darkness being ignorant to the truth of Spirituality.

Religion chose limited answers because it wanted to manipulate the world population in the name of jealousy and competition. Those two feelings not being understood and alchemized are what created religion more than two thousand years ago. All these issues happening in the world today in the name of religion are the residue and last spark of a dying filament from unbalanced jealousy and competitive emotions. All the killing, all the fighting and all the manipulation in the name of religion and religious land being claimed for one culture over the next is a false perspective of our reality. How can anyone claim Mother Earth when we are apart of her and she is apart of us? All she has to do is sneeze and we will all be gone. Our relationship is symbiotic and must be seen as such for the shift to the new paradigm.

I believe the new paradigm is spiritually listening to our truth inside; also called our soul. Yogic philosophy speaks of our soul as the leader of our human experience. The saying, "we are a Spiritual being having a human experience" is a perfect description of how we are meant to perceive life. This is where yogic philosophy fills in the gaps where religion falls short. All my seeking, all my studying and all my focus towards Spirituality led me to discover where we can all meet in the middle, where all of Truth resides. The ancient sages knew this and lived this way. In other words, Magic is Spirituality in motion. Human experience is Magic in manifested motion. That is what I teach in my Kundalini yoga classes and what I have been seeking my whole life.

I believe that is what all the religions attempted to speak about, but during the Piscean Age man lost touch with the native people and ways of seeing things. Therefore, they did not understand the underlying meaning in any of the religious texts and it has gone on for too long. Certain religious people have tried to explain the deeper meaning of these texts for hundreds of years, but not until now were we able to grasp it on a larger scale. It is no mistake that now is the time of this deeper understanding. It is a time that coincides with the awakening of the Age of Aquarius when many people on Earth will begin to wake up. I am one of them and there are many others whose voices have been silenced. We are beginning to understand on a massive scale that to be alive today means we must look within for our answers. That is how quantum physicists are beginning to coincide with the ancient wisdom and knowledge for the rest of humanity on Earth.

Biologists, chemists, doctors and many others have looked at all of our inner anatomy, but now they are researching the infinitely smaller parts that make us up. We are finally ready technologically, medically and scientifically to see atoms and molecules for what they truly are; light vibrations. It is like the saying, "the answer was right under their nose the whole time." Well thanks to people like, Dr. Joe Dispenza and biologist Dr. Bruce Lipton, "Power of Now" and "A New Earth" author

Ekhardt Tolle, "The Five Agreements" author Don Miguel Ruiz and thought minister Michael Beckwith, humanity is beginning to receive the answers from within just as the ancient ones predicted we are meant to be doing.

The way I came to this conclusion about religion being completely different from Spirituality, to which I call living in the magic of life, is apart of my life's journey. I have believed since the age of three when I would ask my aunt, my dad, and my mom to tell me, "why am I here," that I came here for a reason. I suppose some people wonder the same thing, but it most likely does not consume them to the point of creating a life journey for the answers at such a young age, but I truly needed to know. I felt like I knew on some level, but could not remember and the frustration kept me seeking.

I chose to be born into a Jewish family with both parents being Jewish. As my life continued, my mother simultaneously decided she was no longer going to participate in the Jewish authority because as I explained earlier, it was not working for her any longer and the stigma of needing to belong was exhausted. From my understanding, once she began to do her own investigating into other philosophies such as Christian Science, she found what resonated for her. While she was on her journey, I was growing up with no answers to my most important question. Therefore, as I dabbled in every religion on a mission to discover my own answers, my quest was insatiable. Nothing ever resonated with me long enough to feel a quench to my thirst for the truth.

Growing up with my mother after she divorced my father and was a single parent, she asked college students from UCLA to live with us as nannies. We had a girl, Anna, who was Mexican for a while, then came Lulu, she was Chinese and finally I remember Natalie, who was French. I learned as much as I could about their cultures from them and in my young mind their culture equaled their religion. It made sense in my mind that a lifestyle is what a religion attempts to design, but fails to uphold because the foundation was not built on truth.

Around that same time, my biological father was taking me to many AA meetings where their philosophy was based on Christian beliefs to heal their alcoholism. Then in high school, I was fortunate to have my best friend who was Mormon. One summer, I was blessed to stay with her and her family and they took me to their annual summer family camp in Provost, Utah. There, I learned so much about what the Mormons believe, which gave me some answers, but it did not resonate with me enough to convert. There were many things unanswered about what they believed.

I wanted to continue to build upon my experiences and my knowledge to form a clearer answer. It was my world religions class that I found many of the answers about religion that I was seeking at that time. When our professor showed us a diagram of the world religions with a time line, the diagram showed us that the world began as one religion and proceeded to branch off into two religions Eastern and Western. Judaism being the first of all Western religions then turned into Catholicism, Muslim, Christianity, and Mormonism. It was the Eastern religions that really intrigued me at that moment of my life. The Ancient Era included the Kaliyuga, the vedic writings and Hinduism which at the same time in China Confucious began writing in the far East. Finally, from there formed the beginnings of Indian Buddhism,

Chinese Buddhism and Taoism. This provided me with more information and a basis from which to begin a more focused quest for my inner desire.

What is so interesting is that we have no writings or scriptures other than the Vedic scriptures and cave drawings from more than five thousand years ago before organized religion. Although, I have been taught and I have read about the mystical side of almost all religions such as Toltec, Sufism, Kabbalah, and the Brahmans and how their truths were secretly passed down from master to student through story. This would make total sense in explaining why from a logical standpoint that no writings could be found. The mysticism is the Spiritual lifestyle taught through observation from parents and community to the children. The medicine women, crones, sages and ancient ones lived inside this Spiritual knowledge practicing it daily, speaking it to their children and passing on the truth to the fortunate generations.

Therefore, returning to the idea of our world beginning with one religion perhaps points us to all of it being Magic. Call it what you will, but it is mysticism, it is Spirituality and it is the energy of gathering all together to allow Creation a way of expressing itself through us and it must be remembered today. It is very similar to what I have learned about the Native American Indians or the Mayans even, yet still predates even their civilizations. These two civilizations lived with a mentality that they came from "Father Sky and Mother Earth," which I learned from Dr. Bruce Lipton PhD from our Biology of Belief course. He continues saying, "they lived thinking that every thing had a living spirit inside. All the animals, all the blades of grass and all the trees had spirits that they communicated with. They would thank the animal that was going to be killed before they killed it by thanking its spirit before even seeing the animal."

The lifestyle described a practice by these native people from the America's, where everyday was lived as a gift and it resembles a Spiritual perspective, which the ancient yogic philosophy explains too. The yogis in history are the ancient ones who understood all the gifts of the human body and mind that control the elements. How do I know this? I know because in yogic philosophy a true yogi, even today, can control their body's metabolism and central nervous system. When a yogi in India can control their inner nature, they can also control nature outside and around them. In a book I read by Nancy Cooke, titled "Finding Gurus," she tells a story of seeing first hand a yogi transform a cup of water into a frozen block of ice. The yogi goes on to explain to Ms. Cooke that she cannot share this secret with any white people on film because they would abuse the sacred knowledge. This feels not only true to me after practicing yoga for twenty-one years and three of which I have been teaching and practicing Kundalini yoga, but a clear road map for the future of all people living on Earth now and into the future.

As life would have it, while writing this chapter, I went to take a Kundalini yoga class with one of my favorite teachers, Guru Singh this Sunday morning. As it is always a sheer pleasure to be filled up with his energetic field, his knowledge and his experience, being that he is a third generation yogi and Kundalini yogi for most of his life, I was so bold as to ask him for a quote for this chapter. Kindly he agreed, "Everything in existence is Spiritual, choose the highest frequency amongst everything.

That is what is called Spirituality," by Guru Singh. There we have it Earth family.

I will translate this to how I understand it: religion, sports, making love, eating food, school learning, animals, fighting, Iphones, podcasts, cars, the beach and the sun, the moon and the stars are all Spiritual. Are we able to see these things and believe in these things as being apart of everything at its core with a high frequency mindset? Can we speak at our highest vibrational frequency all the time? Can we play sports at our highest frequency? Can we learn at our highest frequency? Can we make love at our highest frequency? I estimate the meaning of this quote to be equivalent to all scientific findings by quantum physicists, neuro-physicists and molecular biologists.

Seeing all of Life as molecules of infinite possibility is one truth that Guru Singh is talking about when seeing everything as Spirituality in motion whether it is a lion, a human, a feeling or the oceans' waves. It is in the ocean's highest frequency to carry the wind and the energy to make its' waves; for if the ocean had no movement, our planet would be very different.

By the way, the quote of living at our highest frequency includes death because death is simply a transformation of energy from living inside a human body to living among all energy outside the human body. I believe this about death to a deep degree. This was confirmed over and over for me ever since my childhood friend died in the beginning of my sophmore year in high school, or when my first grandfather died in 1992 right after my friend or this year when my biological father died. I can share that I did not feel the same way with the first death I experienced as I did to this most recent death of my biological father.

I feel closer to my biological father now that he has transformed than ever. In the same way that I feel like I know Dr. Wayne Dyer better now that he has passed on. I had heard his name when he was alive because of how famous he was, but I never picked up one of his books. Once he was transformed past human form, his words, his essence and his subtle body found me at a time when I was ready. We always feel sad when someone close has passed, but what we are unaware of is that, we can still communicate. Spirituality for me is an understanding of energy and light in my human form and because we are energy and so are the beings passed on, we can actually communicate better. The difference is in the response. It will be through a sign and all we have to do is ask for that sign and be ready to see it.

This understanding of seeing everything as its essence, like a molecule or atom is rather scientific. Therefore, it may be easier to simply say that everything is Spirituality and that we do not need to rely on a pastor or Rabbi to tell us what is spiritual because we will do the work. One way of doing the work is coming to my Kundalini yoga classes, developing a relationship to your Self through your experiences in class and then you will be mindful enough to see every moment as Spiritual.

As I sit here at Kreation café in Santa Monica writing these sentences, I have my earphones in listening to Snatum Kaur, who I got the benefit of seeing in concert last week after being invited by a special soul, while looking across the street to see bougainvillea blowing in the breeze above a barber shop sign flashing, "Open, open...!" This is a perfect moment of me living inside the Spirituality of life. Snatum Kaur is one of the most well known singers of Kundalini mantra music and her music elevates all those that hear it to a Spiritual level. Living in our OPEN hearts and going through our lives is what Guru Singh was talking about because when you are open in your heart, you are vibrating at your highest frequency.

Let me go even deeper into Spirituality by saying that when we are living in this way, we are truly living in the magic of life as this is where it all begins. Once the magic begins through a more spiritual existence, something elevating happens and we begin to develop the most important relationship one can have, which is the relationship with our Infinite Self. For me this is exactly how I see myself living in the magic of life daily. I have developed such a strong relationship with my inner Self, that I have relaxed into my inner Self, being free to create my life moments. My moments are continually surprising and magical because I am in the present being alive and mindful to see the magic unfold.

My life moments that I am sharing with you which I truly consider to be pure magic, all create a specific feeling inside of me. Allowing me to be very precise about the feeling of Spirituality in my life because it contains a feeling never to be mistaken. My feeling during a spiritual moment feels like an overwhelming calmness mixed with an intense exaltation from somewhere in my lower belly all the way up to my heart. A physical signal from my brain sends itself to every cell in my body and a quiet awe takes hold of me until all I can do is cry in pure bliss. It is so uplifting that every time it happens again and again and again, I never want to come back down to any lower frequencies or vibrations and now I don't. I still have moments of challenge, but I believe them to be apart of the magic because they force me to remember to expand and therefore, they are not back at that lower frequency from earlier in my life. Even if every challenge seems difficult, I remember that the magic that will follow the challenge will be more elevating for my mind/body/soul. Then I become excited again and the magic re-appears right in front of my eyes.

    Spirituality and the spiritual journey becomes like waiting for waves to crash on the shore or a fireworks show. We are never sad that a wave is smaller than the last. We enjoy the sound of the wave and we are ever impatient for the next one to crash upon the shore. Nor are we disappointed when a red firework goes off and then a purple firework following even if we were hoping for all the fireworks to be red ones. We are simply impressed and excited by the beauty that continues to explode in front of our eyes. Spirituality teaches us through every moment that we must maintain that omnipresent anticipation for what is to come because no matter the current challenge or moment, we are grateful to be apart of it all. Yogi Bhajan said, "Spirituality is the whole ocean and you were one drop of water within the whole ocean."

    Adding my own piece of opinion onto Yogi Bhajan's quote, I will yet again share a final story about how Spirituality works in my life as magic. Soon after I arrived home from writing this chapter, I found myself alone with my two young sons. They were at a moment where they needed to calm down a bit. So, I turned on Netflix to get a kids movie like Trolls or Sing, but I found The Prophet. I had never been able to finish reading the book because when I was younger it always seemed to be metaphorical writing. For the first time, I understood the whole book and both of my boys watched most of the film with me, which is pretty incredible for four year and seventeen month young kids. The visuals are stunning, the art is stunning, and the voices are wonderful all of which facilitate a clear understanding of Khalil Gibran's writing. "I love when you bow in your mosque, kneel in your temple, pray in your church. For you and I are sons of one religion, and it is the spirit," Khalil Gibran. All of life is a Spiritual ocean if we could have the eyes to see that we are constantly swimming within it...

Meditation:
Releasing Childhood Anger

This meditation will give you some subtle powers and it will change you inside and out.

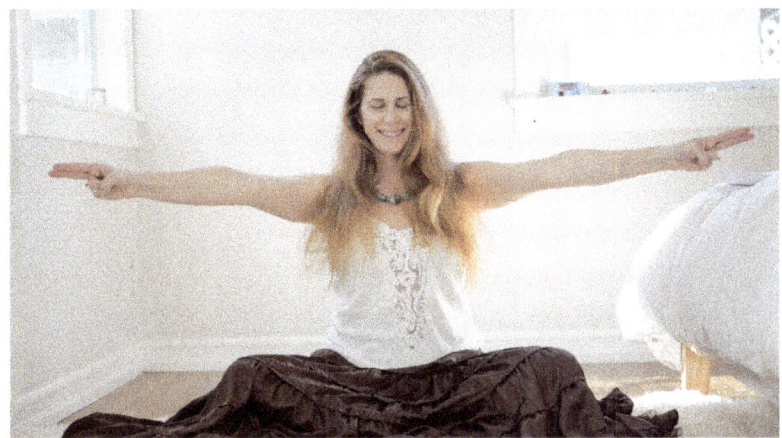

Sit in easy pose with your arms outstretched to the sides. No bend in the elbows and you use your thumbs to lock down the Mercury and Sun fingers while you extend the Jupiter and Saturn fingers. Palms face forward with fingers out to the sides. Begin to deeply breathe by sucking air through your closed teeth and exhale through your nose.

Do this for 11 minutes and to finish: inhale deeply, hold the breath for 10 seconds while you stretch your spine up with arms out to the sides. Exhale and repeat two more times.

If done in the evening, you will find that your whole caliber and energy is changed the next morning.

Chapter 9

Experiences With Unexplainable Energy

"Everything is energy and that's all there is to it. Match the frequency of the reality you want and you cannot help but get that reality. It can be no other way. This is not philosophy. This is physics."
    -Albert Einstein

"The energy of the mind is the essence of life."
    -Aristotle

"If you want to find the secrets of the universe, think in terms of energy, frequency and vibration…"
    -Nikola Tesla

This chapter is a pivotal chapter for Living in the Magic of Life because today is a special day for you energetically if you have gotten this far in the book. Some experiences I will share in this chapter are to be taken as a new magical criterion for all of us in our lives. This is my intention. I have asked my guides to lead me up a road, which will cease to be merely me sharing my experiences, ideas and opinions because it will be my guides pulling my past experiences out of my memory for you to assimilate it. These energy stories will become an exemplary road to reach you where you are at in your life's journey with everything you have experienced. If you can relate to any part of my stories and use them for your own life to grow and feel centered in relation to what you have experienced on your life journey.

As I have requested, my guides are leading both you and me to travel through a wormhole of time and space where our beliefs of energy and magic will be forever changed. Together we will co-create a new perspective as this is the way to expand. As my guides light up this wormhole tunnel, one foot in front of the other, I will lay out the stories as I discover them for you to see. I am becoming well versed in the inter-dimensional lifestyle that resides subtly between the energetic unseen world, society's world and my inner world.

First, I am using mind energy to flow towards you in your life through writing the words so that you will begin to float higher in your personal energy field and vibrate at a higher frequency. This energy is my electro-magnetic field touching yours via these words and the energy surrounding the electro-magnetic field of this book. Perhaps it feels very similar to when once in your life you have been waiting at a stoplight and you feel something pulling you to turn your head. You look towards the car next to you and the driver has been staring at you. You felt their energy touching your energy. While reading this chapter, you may feel my energy pulling you higher and maybe your brain will tingle or you will feel different. Be protected knowing you are safe even when it feels different. That is how the energy which, I refer to in my book as Magic, might begin to really work for you in your life.

Energy begins to expand once it becomes noticed because energy loves company. We rarely ever talk about energy as something to gauge within our body vessel, let alone enhance it. Our normal conversations are whether we feel we have energy or have no energy that particular day, but this method of measure is no longer accurate for us humans. The truth is, we always have energy, but perhaps if we are feeling low energy or depressed we need to make a shift in our momentary prana or breathing so that our chakra system is not acting stagnant.

If you could so kindly begin to focus on the energy inside your body right now to understand what I am describing in this chapter. Think about the energy you had when you woke up, you used energy to get out of bed, but did you feel excited before you got up? Perhaps, you are about to have an amazing day and the mental energy of that got you up, rather than an alarm. Then you went to make your breakfast and you put your focus and love on the meal you were to prepare. Then the pranic food went into your body giving you energy to get ready for your day and continue to function on a high level. All this energy has gone through you and around you without much effort; just as your heart beats with asking you to help. Or perhaps you had much difficulty getting out of bed, eating and preparing for your day because a life challenge is weighing on you. What if you could help yourself cultivate a more powerful energetic life experience to give your body and mind energy all the time?

Imagine that you could jump out of bed with an excitement so profound, you practically lifted off your bed like a space shuttle. You fly into your kitchen to make your coffee or tea and as your turn on the TV or your phone, a song titled, "Best Day of My Life" comes on. Then you float into your closet and the exact outfit pops out at you and you can add your creative personal touch with a pair of socks or a scarf depending on your creativity for that day. The rest of your day plays out in this manner where everything is in perfect place, songs come onto the radio wherever you are that start to speak to you in every moment. Finally, imagine this possibility one step further extending throughout your entire year as your life begins to flourish into infinite possibility exploding in front of your eyes just like this day. This is what scientists call Quantum Physics by you living in the motion of possibility. If you read Anita Moorjani's book, "Dying To Be Me," you will hear her version of how we must look at our own lives.

In this moment, my mental energy is so charged by this wormhole doorway that I am standing in that I am able to notice the energy all around me feeling alive as it spins. It is lifting me up so that my body and my mind feel like they are super charged. I have a flow of supportive ideas and I can lift my attitude so that the energy surrounding me becomes prosperous. I attract the people I am supposed to meet today. I have conversations that revolve around the subject of my book or things that I have been curious about for the last few months. It is the Magic supporting this book and the energy around that support bringing us through this wormhole to another paradigm where this new life is possible for all of us.

I am aware inside of this wormhole now how the Magic is bringing me up to where the cosmic power wants us to go. I have been open to Magic, craving it actually, for a very long time since I began experiencing little spurts of enhanced energy sprinkled throughout my life. As you can tell if you have been reading this book since the beginning, I had my first experience of powerfully enhanced energy at an Aura-soma shop. It took me a long time to recover from that experience, but I stayed connected and open at a distance to the belief that energy of that magnitude was worth revisiting. I have some more stories to share that helped me begin to solidify a consistent curiosity towards energy being the only universal truth.

Before I begin sharing my stories, I would like to also expand your mind and/or perspective by asking you to think about the Internet for a moment. When the Internet was first available to anyone outside of the Military, I was in middle school and it was called the World Wide Web. Those three words are so accurate because they refer to web of energy and how we are all connected within the web just like the Internet has the ability to connect us through the seemingly invisible space. Dr. Bruce Lipton calls the web, a matrix like in the movie, The Matrix. Yogi Bhajan called it two things, the Aura and the Electro-magnetic field. The truth is our world does have a matrix, an aura or a field, but so do our bodies. Our aura is our electro-magnetic web that radiates out from within our being, like an energy source.

When I was in seventh grade, I used to spend a lot of time at friends' houses. My best friend at the time had a computer and she had the Internet. Her father worked as an engineer with computers and she had one of the first laptops I had ever seen and she taught me how to use AOL to "chat" with boys from different states. It felt so exhilarating to flirt across states in real time. I couldn't have predicted at my young age in seventh grade the speed of advancement with which computers and the Internet would take, but I knew I was hooked. Of course if I loved it that much, than so would everyone on our planet. The World Wide Web has truly become a phenomenon of our times.

I use the Internet everyday all day long sometimes whether for work or pleasure. I have gotten to the point where I must limit myself using the World Wide Web because I realize that despite what it provides, it takes me away from my innate ability to connect with people in front of me in the moment. What is even better now is that computers cost hundred of dollars less than when they were first sold commercially. We have computers on our phones and we in essence have answers at our fingertips.

I've heard and read by many who agree that the 19th century was the industrial revolution and that the 20th century is the informational revolution. The amazing notion about the informational revolution happening now is how it allows us to connect from further away. We are able to learn, to socialize, to know and to connect instantly to the other side of the planet, thanks to the Internet. Although this is exceptional, I find myself wondering why has our collective destiny brought us to this?

This destiny or path is clearly no mistake, especially if we look at what steps the world took to get us to this day and time. History tells us we fought with each other for thousands of years killing each other over power or independence from the people in power. Subsequently, during the last hundred years, we began working together, to industrialize ourselves. It definitely paid off, as there are less third world countries than even fifty years ago and we're not killing ourselves in wars as before. More and more countries are catching up with a world standard in technology and in industry than ever before. Technology is continuing to expand ever rapidly now that we have introduced the Internet, but we forget that this has spanned less than twenty-five years. Therefore, we must be meant to be going in this direction as a human race to progress our species.

The reason has occurred to me recently, as I discovered how to use energy within myself, that all of this is because when we can learn to connect with each other across the world through the Internet, soon after we will understand that we are all connected without the Internet, too. Basically people will begin to understand that their actions and behaviors have an effect on others across the world because we are all truly apart of the web of life. We will feel the energy emanating within our beings from the other side of the world. Perhaps the Internet will even teach us to use our innate gifts of mental telepathy, clairsentience, clairvoyance, intuition, premonition, telekinesis, and even walking through walls.

At the very least, the Internet is infusing us with more compassion as we can see the earthquakes, tsunamis, and hurricanes happening in real time. I remember watching for the first time in Thailand when their 2004 tsunami hit exactly what Mother Earth does with her power and how much love welled up inside of me for all the people affected. It affected everyone to see a natural disaster in real time. Then came hurricane Katrina, then, was the volcano in Iceland that erupted and literally halted air travel over Europe for a month. Then was the horrible Earthquake in Japan followed by their Tsunami and I was literally able to see the Tsunami coming as it was in real time, thanks to the Internet and CNN. This year alone we've witnessed Houston, Saint Barth and Puerto Rico. Simply renaming all these disasters is enough for me to be convinced that what happens on our planet affects every person. Mother Earth is speaking up and we must begin to listen.

    I recently discovered a female American scientist living in England who is using energy at a distance to heal people's diseases from across the world through intentions or prayers such as Shamans do for their communities. Her name is Lynn McTaggert. She has a large following that she leads in a global intention focused on healing one person she chose for that day. She has found that it works and she writes about her findings in a book entitled, The Field. Then she published a new book based on findings from other scientists, physicists, biologists and psychologists who confirm our true energetic connection with one another in, "The Bond."

    "The Bond," talks about our connection to everyone and everything in the world and the bond we innately share just like I spoke about earlier with the web and matrix of life. Lynn basically says that all beings have a need to help one another rather than compete against. She continues, " we are inescapably connected, hardwired to each other at our most elemental level- from cells to whole societies." Upon reading this blurb, I believe it confirms that our evolutionary direction alongside the Internet is towards an awakening to our elemental essence of energy use to heal one another, to interact one another and to evolve next to one another.

Science is always changing and even this face is based on Quantum Physics because if we humans observe something and can change the outcome to create different possibilities than, we will forever be creating new truths and this is the Magic I am referring to throughout. After a few years, most of the well-known scientists from now will be surpassed by new research in science just like Darwin's theory on evolution being found false or even Einstein's discovery on the law of the photoelectric effect. The elements of their research were "stepping stones" for the scientists of tomorrow. Of course we all agree that those men were quite brilliant, but just as life evolves so do its' scientists. Let us become our own scientist testing Magic and our own energy to create the future at the highest frequency imaginable.

Now let's get into some stories. Remember these stories are simply examples for you to use if you like and how you like. My first experience with powerful energy happened one morning. I spent the night with a friend from work in Santa Monica near the beach. I was working at Geoffrey's in Malibu, California and a guy had become a good friend of mine.

We went up to his roof because he had a gorgeous view of the Pacific Ocean. A great conversation was in full animation about life and Quantum Physics as I began to lift my frequency and my mind up. As we continued philosophizing about all the possibilities in life I began to go into another dimension. I still present to our conversation, but I ceased to be attached to my thoughts or anything outside of my body.

As we looked towards the beach to watch the ocean dance with the wind, we noticed a large group of crows dancing in flight. The longer we watched the more I let go until I had a feeling about the crows that was a stereotype from society. I expressed to him that I was not so fond of crows because I thought they signified death. Immediately as I finished explaining my aversion to the black birds, we watched a crow get struck by an electrical current from a telephone pole. The crow fell dead to the roof top underneath.

We were both shocked with our mouths gaping open unable to speak or make sense out of it. Neither of us had ever seen that type of thing before and when we did finally begin to voice what we had seen it was unnerving for us both. I could not help but wonder if I had done that somehow; by my story or by my energy with the realization that I maybe did leave for another dimension. In any case, on a deep level, I knew we had done that somehow.

I went on with my life without any research or questioning into that occurrence with the crow and continued following life's flow. A few years later, I had returned from France on yet another vacation trip. I went to a Hollywood party up in the hills of Laurel Canyon by myself. Everyone going to the party had to take a bus from a parking area to the mansion where the party was happening. The party was uneventful for me as I was sober at that time and only knew the two party promoters. Everyone was drinking and trying to be seen as a Hollywood movie star or wannabe.

As I was leaving the party one guy Sylvain began talking to me. It turned out that he was French. I thought in that moment that he must have picked up on the French vibe I was giving off; having recently returned from the Cote d'Azur. I began to speak to him in French and we proceeded to have a "real" conversation. He and I both felt major chemistry and we rode down the hill to our cars together. I gave him my number thinking we would see each other soon.

After a few months, I had not heard from Sylvain, but I continued to do the Hollywood actress thing of auditioning, acting classes, and creating networking to help my career advance at that time. I was invited to a friend's movie set on Venice Beach where he was filming his first major film. While I was there, I thought of Sylvain and called him randomly. I did not reach him, but I left him a message. He called me back a few hours later saying that he was leaving on a plane that day to go to Paris and that he would call me back upon his arrival.

When he called me back a few weeks later, I was so excited and we made a date to go out. He told me that he was taking me to a movie wrap party, (which is when a movie is finished being filmed and the production team celebrates.) Coincidently or not, Sylvain took me to my friends wrap party, the same friend who was filming at Venice Beach the day I called Sylvain who was on a plane to Paris. I was so surprised at the syncronicity and so excited to be out with this handsome man. The pure hilariousness of these two lives intermixing at this wrap party was giving me elated cells and my heart began to feel enchanted. That moment began to remind me of the time I spent in Cannes at Film Festival from a few years before. As Sylvain and I began to leave the wrap party to get some food down the street, it began to rain.

We walked close together down the street and he held me into his body. We passed by three different valet stands where the valet guys were waiting for patrons to arrive. Every valet stand we passed with no explanation I could imagine, their umbrellas began to spring open all by themselves, one after the next. The final and third umbrella literally almost hit me in the head as if to say your energy is powerfully moving us. I have never been sure if Sylvain even noticed, but I certainly did because I felt the energy do it and when I looked to see if the valet guy had done anything, they were as shocked as me. Sylvain and I never talked about it, but it certainly sparked a deeper curiosity within me about how I did that.

I continued to date Sylvain and almost every time I saw him, I felt that elated feeling. I began to manifest the most amazing experiences with him, but I could never fully understand how to use that exalted energy under my control. For example, I continued to see lights switch off and on when we were kissing and I remember wishing to understand how to harness that energy. My relationship with Sylvain never developed into something important, but those experiences with energy was another foreshadow into my future.

It wasn't until recently that I realized I needed subconscious cleaning from all the childhood programming that I awakened to healing myself on a deeper level. Now, I am starting to use my energy in a more informed and controlled potential. It is due to all the Kundalini yoga and meditation I do that allows me to clarify the questions about energy I have always asked. I am getting back to the point of total comprehension of all the cumulative life experiences, which have always been pointing me in the direction of Magical living forever. The energy of magic is pushing me through the wormhole tunnel of Life towards living only magical occurrences, experiences and true heaven on Earth for all of us so that we begin use the energy always available to us.

Meditation:
Regulate the Systems of the Body

This meditation is to re-organize the communication to every organ and regulate the body for calming. It can improve menopause problems and glandular system problems.

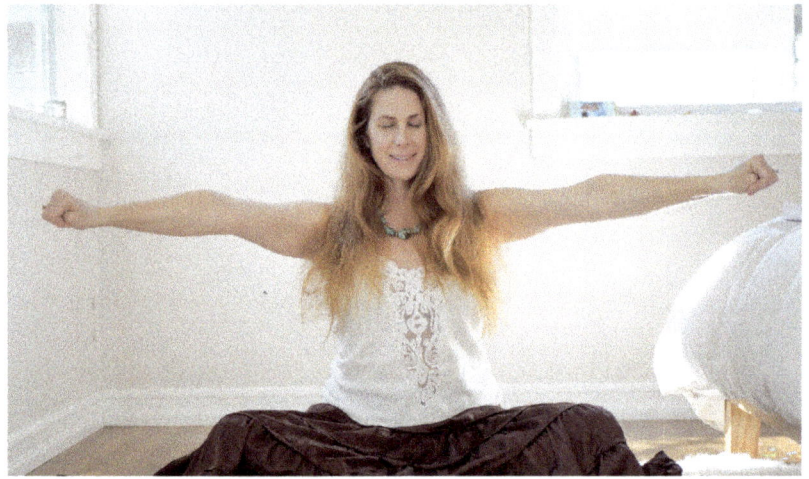

Sit in easy pose with spine straight. Stretch arms out to the sides with the palms down. Touch the thumbs from each hand to the mound under the Mercury finger. Close your fists over the thumbs.

As you maintain straight elbows, begin to row backwards in 18 inch circles.

The breath is like a hiss inhale and exhale through the nose. You must pull the air in and out by squeezing the nostrils to make the hiss sound.

Moving quickly to the music, "Tantric Har" has the rhythm to keep you going.

To finish: deeply fill the rib cage with air and hold for 8 seconds. Exhale powerfully through the mouth like a cannon fire and repeat this sequence two more times.

Chapter 10

Love and Miracles

"A miracle is a shift in perception from fear to love."
    -Marianne Williamson

"Where there is great love there are always miracles."
    -Willa Cather

"Miracles happen everyday, change your perception of what a miracle is and you'll see them all around you."
    -Jon Bon Jovi

At this point I would like to pull you through the wormhole with me, too because I am passionate about love. If I am going to stand here in awe of our world, in awe of our energetic capacities as humans and in awe of our future, above all the darkness, I might as well share it with you like-minded people. I believe we are all like-minded people because we are all humans. Therefore, I will proceed with another deep question: What if miracles are not miracles at all? What if they are simply thoughts that became possible and manifested into view right before our eyes. We would no longer believe that our thoughts were impossible sounds no one can hear but us. What if anything is truly possible?

My whole life up to now has shown me that miracles exist and I am finally saying along with Yogi Bhajan that, "I rely on miracles." Instead of saying they may exist, I say they have become apart of my normal existence. Can miracles become normal for everyone? They are simply the Magic of Life existing right before our eyes in every moment. Eventually, you can look up at the sky to see the color blue with the puffy white clouds blowing in the wind and say to yourself, even this is a miracle.

Therefore, if you can see the simplest thing and re-imagine it as a miracle, then your mind will begin to see and create miracles everywhere. You will call miracles of all kinds into your daily life, from being invited to a concert you have wanted to attend for a long time to a meeting your favorite celebrity to getting a parking spot right in front of where you are going to why not millions of dollars in your bank if that is the kind of miracle you need. The word miracle holds an energetic vibration that shifts our mental tuning into a higher vibration. That is the energetic law of our reality with words; the symbols of communication, like Don Miguel Ruiz explains in his book, "The Four Agreements." All we have to do is lather ourselves up with the word, miracle, by repeating it over and over until our subconscious mind learns to see miracles as our true human existence.

I can begin listing all the miracles in my life that I thought at one time were impossible, but now I realize I was simply ignorant. It was false to think that way because I forgot like most of us that I am a miracle. If you think about it, we are all miracles. Life is a gift and therefore, being born IS a true miracle. If we see everything as miraculous, we are simply living from one miracle to the next. Remember I am sharing this information at a time when the current paradigm is shifting, which should make reading these words easier to believe.

Let us remember the hieroglyphics written on rock walls in caves telling us of the past ways of life. Are those not miraculous for the human race to be able to see? From my perspective, it is miraculous that we have even survived since before those writings. Furthermore it is as if humans were MEANT to evolve from then until now exactly as we have and even further into the future. It's incredible that human nature and the need to share our existence has not changed since cave men were writing on walls. We still crave to share about our lives, just as our ancestors did back inside those caves. (That is what I was craving as a reason to write this book. Partly to get my messages out to see if anyone has lived some of the same things and partly because I had the need to tell someone all of this.) Again, is that not super miraculous that we, you, me and everyone, are somehow related to those cave men, even though it feels like that is impossible somehow? Let us now make a pact with ourselves to change our perspectives and our beliefs to remember to let more miracles reveal themselves easily one after the next.

A miraculous experience that I would like to share which proved to me that miracles are an everyday phenomenon and must be implemented into the psyche of the human race moving forward. Perhaps I am not the only one who believes miracles are normal, but then let us begin talking about it out in our world. Let us begin the conversation in our daily lives, homes, neighborhoods and communities instead of talking about the weather. If I start, perhaps others will join me and then every person will join us until the most important conversation becomes only about how many miracles occurred for us in a given day. Then, our children will have this perspective as an opportunity to help them be happy and win in their own lives. This is what it will take to shift the paradigm and either we can go against it, like swimming up a rapid river, or we go with the flow within the current paradigm shift. Can we evolve or die?

That miraculous experience from ten years ago, which I never told anyone had happened until now will stay in my memory forever. I was visiting my sister at her store on Montana Ave. in Santa Monica. All of a sudden we heard a car screech to a stop super loud up the street. Next, we heard a man screaming at the top of his lungs with a cry so scary it would probably not be repeatable from a sound department in a sound studio for movies. Something inside me pushed me to run outside to see. As I ran into the street, I was being pushed to run and see exactly what was happening. When I arrived to the street corner a half block up, I found a child being held by his mother. I was one of three humans to arrive in the middle of the street at this boy's side. His mother was hysterically crying saying he had been hit by the car that was stopped with the man screaming outside his car.

The boy had no shoes on and he had been hit so hard, it pushed him to fly into the air about twenty feet forward away from the crosswalk. He was unconscious and not moving at all. People were yelling to call an ambulance and the police. Other onlookers from all the stores had walked out to this horrifically sad sight. Something inside me told me to put my hands on this boy's shoulders. So, I touched his feet and I began to pray in my mind and send love energy into his body. As I started to open my mind for directions to flow in to guide me, my mind became like a vacuum and all thought had been sucked right out. I was left with miraculous emptiness.

It was just like in the movies where everything slows down and the scene becomes clear for the main character. I held onto the toddlers' tiny feet, holding them until something could come through me and into him. After three minutes, the boy began to cry and the now crowd all around us, also began to cry as if they were all holding their breath with him. Whatever had taken place inside of me was surprising and at that time in my reality I did not comprehend what had happened. Right after the boy began to cry, the fire trucks arrived with ambulances. I took a moment to look up and exit my meditative, channeled state. A fireman arrived and instinctually I stood up to make a place for him to kneel down next to the boy. I slowly walked back to my sister's store and acted like nothing had happened to me because I couldn't explain such a miracle in that minute. Inside myself somewhere, I felt a clear knowing about what had just occurred.

As I continue to study with scientists, physicists, neurologists and as a Kundalini yoga student and teacher, I am beginning to hear the dialog more and more that we humans must shift our perspective and open to love as an actual energy. As Dr. Darren Weisman, who works with the "Life Line Method" of healing, says, "once we shift what we look at, what we see begins to shift." He and Dr. Bruce Lipton have spoken about miracles and how scientifically "if you believe something in your mind, the outside reality must create the images and circumstances in reality." Therefore, perhaps like Jesus, once you believe you can walk on water or hot coals, you will see it materialize in front of your eyes. Or perhaps for a more approachable example, if you believe you are already with the love of your life, he/she will appear.

Let us open to love as a means to understand miracles with our hearts and not our minds. Love energy exudes as more of a feeling inside the body and the neutral mind. It is almost like an effervescence that energizes us to live in the light especially when it is fresh and new. That is why falling in love leads one to go inside the ENERGY of love. Upon "falling" in love with another human, whether an adult or a baby, we believe we feel better when with that other person and because we believe it, we do feel better. This feeling of falling in love with someone else is simply the introduction to love energy or energy. There are levels of understanding that occur for humans to evolve out of ignorance and into the next level. The next level of love energy is falling in love with oneself, which further evolves us into living in the Magic of Life. The next to last level is when we fall in love with all of life and that is the ultimate love energy. It is this love energy that vibrates at the frequency of the universe and creates magical thinking and miraculous living.

Once this type of love energy has been experienced it becomes a way of seeing all of life and we can live in love energy all the time. The goal is always magical living though, how you get there will be different for each person. Depression can become a thing of the past. Sadness can become a thing of the past. Darkness can become a thing of the past. If you can walk to the top of Mt. Everest and see the whole world from above, you can never un-see that. When you return to sea level and you understand where you have been and what you have seen on the journey, you have started the shift into Living in the Magic of Life.

My metaphor example of climbing the ladder of love energy levels explains my experience of how it happened for me when I met my husband. I knew I wanted to perfect my French skills and going to work in France over the summer between my junior and senior year at University was my solution. I had no preconceived plan to go to France, meet the love of my life and live happily every after. I simply put myself into my dreams of living in France and being fluent in that language. The miracle happened when I saw the bar tender, Mika, from far away that first day visiting my family's favorite beach club. I have heard that luck is simply a mix of preparation dancing with opportunity. It was as though some invisible karmic string was pulling us together. I felt so strongly interested in him, but I did not understand why. Because I was dating another guy, I resisted that intuitional pull towards Mika. It was lucky, but I tried to put him out of my mind. Mika must have felt an invisible attraction deeply as well because he thought of our meeting as lucky, too. He has told me all these years later that he had to break past his resistance of timidity to even talk to me that first night after work.

We have been together for eighteen years and we have discussed our initial meeting multiple times. He says he had noticed me before my first night of work, as well. What got him to push past his deep lifelong handicap of shyness was that the first night he asked me to come hang out with him, I did not. He made it his mission to ensure the following night we would have time together and the second night he got his wish. Oddly, I did, too, and I have all this time since. It was the best decision we both decided to pursue because we have both evolved so much from the relationship.

Mika is my love miracle because he was the vehicle that helped me discover the ladder of love energy. It was my learning through living that gave me the desire to explore my inner world during this whole relationship. He brings something so immeasurable and vast out of me still. I believe that our relationship can only be characterized as karmic or past life mate. Since falling in love with him eighteen years ago, our love has taught me about love energy with all its colors and emotions.

I found my inner scientist pushing me to discover what love was and why it feels so amazing and yet so painful. Upon the discovery, I was introduced to the first rung of the love energy ladder. I had to explore my feelings more deeply to conclude some answers. I am a clairsentient and I feel love energy deeply. I realized my absorption into that feeling needed to be transmuted so that I could live a life feeling much less co-dependent on another human for my sanity. So, early on in our relationship the feeling of being in love took me so far as to write and to produce a documentary entitled, "Does True Love Really Exist?"

This was before going to NYFA. The documentary shifted into a film idea based on my findings, but I never finished writing the movie because I was still answering the inner questions, until now.

My love for Mika has brought such an intense opening out of me, I felt like anything was possible and I had to learn about those feelings to get to the next rung of evolution. What I learned through the process of choosing to stay in our relationship after every turn taught me about life as a byproduct. I learned about love relationships, which led to me learning to love myself. Through learning to love and accept myself beyond dark emotions, mistakes or self-critiques, I was led to discover the science of quantum physics and neuroplasticity, which was the next rung on the ladder.

When we comprehend the infinite potential (quantum physics) of love for our Self, then the ability to forgive becomes possible. It is our ability to forgive ourselves that leads us to the final rung. Our brain learns that infinite possibilities are simply about learning to live in the LOVE ENERGY constantly in order to create our infinite potential. This love for oneself lasts longer than the honeymoon affect in any relationship, which usually happens in a new relationship during the first six months to one year.

Dr. Bruce Lipton calls it "the honeymoon affect" and he explains what we all feel when we fall in love. It is a feeling of becoming lighter as though we were a bird flying high and seeing all the new beauty we have never seen before. Perhaps feeling as if we are able to do anything, go anywhere with that person and it will feel magical. This kind of love is the infinite well of emotion that one ignites within upon falling in love the first time. It ignites an inner energy so powerful that we feel as if we could lift a car with our bare hands. This inner power or energy during the beginning of the relationship is what Dr. Bruce Lipton, Dr. Darren Weisman and many others refer to as an experience of belief in Self.

This feeling of believing in ourselves so deeply that we never get sick, or that we can spend the whole night awake talking to our lover and then go to work the next day without even batting an eyelash is the first feeling of intense love energy that can change us. I believe it is experienced first with another person and then we must learn to transfer that capacity to our (inner) self. Once, we develop that empowering feeling of self-belief towards our life, than we can enhance it deeper and deeper. The curiosity of falling in love with our inner self, that Self that is Infinite, is the last level of our evolutional ladder. It is where the Living in the Magic of Life was born for me.

Yogi Bhajan said, "People who love are happy." He put it very simply, but it is true and so profound. Once you can discover the deep love for yourself, by Yogi Bhajan's thinking, you can be happy all the time. In my experience, deep Self-love attempts to explain a confidence inside our hearts that says anything is possible and creates a connection to all of Life. This is miraculous Infinity and infinity is within each and every one of us.

During the time when I was first beginning to learn how to fall in love with myself, I had to break up with Mika a few times. One of the last times I broke up with him we were separated for almost two years and Mika was in France while I was in Los Angeles. He had a life threatening car accident where he fell asleep at four a.m. after work and crashed into a tree. The doctors removed his spleen and put him in a medicated coma because of all his head injuries. I was awoken by my stepfather at six a.m. LA time with this news. I thought I would die and when I spoke to Mika's mother she told me not to come unless I planned on staying. She was worried "it would be too challenging for him to have me come and leave again."

I was being tested at the same time he was deciding if he would stay alive or pass on forever. Did I love him enough to commit to him or did I love myself enough to commit to my individual growth. Those three weeks of his coma were heart wrenching for me. I had to make sure he was going to survive, but I had to do it for afar. I kept my presence around the idea that he would be fine, even through the sadness. When he woke up and they determined that he would stay alive the biggest relief came over me. Even if I would not yet make a decision to go and be with him, at least I knew he was somewhere alive and I had the possibility of seeing him again.

After he re-learned to talk, walk and move we stayed in touch. He could not remember everything, but he remembered us and he was sad that we were not together. Nine months later we saw each other in person for the first time since the accident. He picked me up from my grand parents vineyard wearing white pants and a white shirt. He looked like a saint. I was wearing a black dress to be the perfect yin to his yang.

He took me to a restaurant on the top of a mountain that over looked my grand parents vineyard on one side and the Mediterranean Sea on the other side. We sat down at a beautiful table outside with just the right amount of sun next to a wall garden. We did not stop looking at each other for the first thirty minutes. All around us butterflies flew and flowers were blowing in the breeze. It is a moment in my mind that will forever stand still as a magical moment in our lifetime love affair.

We could not deny the immense feeling of magic we both felt that day. It was as if we had a new first meeting because we were new people. The two years we lived separate helped us to grow up in our own ways respectively. He told me all about his accident and the hospital experience, which all changed him on a deep level. I was able to be present in the moment for him. Therefore, after our second "first date" we both walked away feeling fulfilled to have reconnected. Six months later he flew to Los Angeles to "visit" me and during that visit, he proposed. It was such a surprise and he gave me the space to feel the magic and decide what I wanted.

Living in the Magic of Life requires the understanding and wisdom of the love energy levels of going from loving another to loving ourself. Using that ladder as a time for metamorphosis into the butterfly for every individual will create a healthier relationship inside your mind. Becoming the butterfly is being the best version of our Self everyday. Once we have seen that version, we can live life surrounded with the miracles that come with infinite self-love and the enduring perspective change that emanates out as a strong electro-magnetic field. Life becomes a continual flowing river of love energy constantly pushing us to go deeper into that emotion of confidence and love. All the relationship challenges we face in any relationship, all the emotional challenges we face as a human, and all the challenges that life presents to us during our lifetime becomes an opportunity to grow more in love with our inner light. Then one day, after much cultivation of the light, all that is left is the energy of love and then we can transform back into Infinite energy.

This love energy carries us through human life. I believe the correct reference is cloud nine? When we are living on a cloud, we are living in our self-created heaven on Earth. Any health problems are immediately transmuted and we are strong despite any symptoms of doubt. Further, our symptoms become signs for us to look deeper into our self-love and help us to heal stronger to maintain our heavenly life.

I am currently healing stronger after a diagnosis of an auto immune dis-order called Hashimoto Dis-ease. After my abortion in 2009, I was deep in the pain of emotions and had no idea of my Auto Immune challenge, but exactly a year and a half later another miracle occurred as I was led to discover a symptom. A wonderful French gynecologist took her time with me following three miscarriages. She was ahead of most of even American gynecologists because she pushed to discover the dis-order through blood work that was to lead me further on my journey towards my destiny.

Upon seeing my results, she knew who to refer me to so that I could achieve my goal of becoming a mother. She had served her purpose and played a role in pushing me forward towards my destiny. Once Mika and I had the doctor who would perform the IVF work, it was on the first time of doing IVF that I knew everything was on the mend. I was constantly being led by the Magic of Life and I trusted it to help me pick up the breadcrumbs with ever piece of new information. That inner knowing is what has led to my self-healing of the auto immune symptoms that Hashimoto brings up. This auto immune challenge has led to more awareness of my physical body, my nutrition and my mind.

Perhaps if it was not for the difficult health challenge, I would never have re-discovered Kundalini yoga.

The awareness of my thoughts that I had developed through years of Power yoga and self help books allowed me to realize that I had foggy brain and it was not simply being tired with a new baby. Even with a foggy brain, I stayed in the energy of Love that first year of my first son's life and that love energy supported me. I found a doctor that knew how to jump-start my self-healing. He got me on a natural medicine and other brain supplements that supported my healing journey. The fog parted from my brain and I woke up to a richer life providing me more energy of love and self-awareness. Living without the foggy brain helped me to see what I needed to support me in finding the next tool to fix the auto immune dis-order.

Three months before Weston turned two, I found the Kundalini yoga manuels that a friend had given me years before. I knew deep inside that I needed to cure my auto immune challenges and there was an intuitive voice that spoke, telling me to practice Kundalini yoga. Practicing this form of yoga not only provided me experiences of feeling good, it helped me to become clear my mind. I had a new sense of direction, more energy and more motivation to advance into creating love in myself, for my child and for my husband. I began teaching immediately because I fell in love with the feeling this new yoga gave me every time I practiced. As I have heard many times, if you want to master something, you must teach it and I became passionate. Teaching this form of yoga fulfills me because sharing the technology leads me to help others have a better life.

I was driving today and I watched a young woman cross the street in front of my car. I could feel her desire to be seen and accepted by the clothes she was wearing and the way she was walking, but more than that the energy she was giving off. The technology of Kundalini yoga and the yogic philosophy that feeds the practice is the ultimate love energy miracle. It provides a powerful inner connection and self-confidence for me and my students every time we practice. Watching that girl, I remember feeling like I had to dress a certain way to be "accepted," but now I love myself so deeply that I have shifted that old story, thanks to Kundalini yoga and meditation.

I have, yet again, a new perspective on Life and the self love is the cohesive that makes all of my daily experiences miracles; even the challenging ones. I accept myself more after all the experiences I have had in my yoga practice. As I become more acutely aware, my perspective continues to uplift. I can feel my clairsentience being enhanced and becoming like a super power rather than a curse or something that I do not understand which, hinders me from feeling good. I have found a space in life where I can take my time to feel the self love and gauge anything Life may test. I am strong enough to handle the growing stress and stimulation that our society inherently produces as well.

I have created a protective light around me with the discovery of deep self-love from my life experiences. This protective being is my companion. I can rely on this self-love to take over whenever I need it and all I have to do is connect inside. It is this connection and inner conversation that creates the healing, the self-love and the miracle needed in our shifting civilization from the old paradigm to the new. I feel prepared for anything and everything because of this inner confidence that gets strengthened everyday. Therefore, instead of living in fear I have shifted my inner mantra to "how can I love these challenges and emotions for providing me new experiences to practice self-love?" My days are one long yoga class filled with breathing, stretching, challenging moments and total relaxation into letting go into Self Love.

Meditation:
Removing Fear of the Future

This meditation takes away your fears of the future, which have been created by your subconscious memories of the past. It will force you to deal with your heart center.

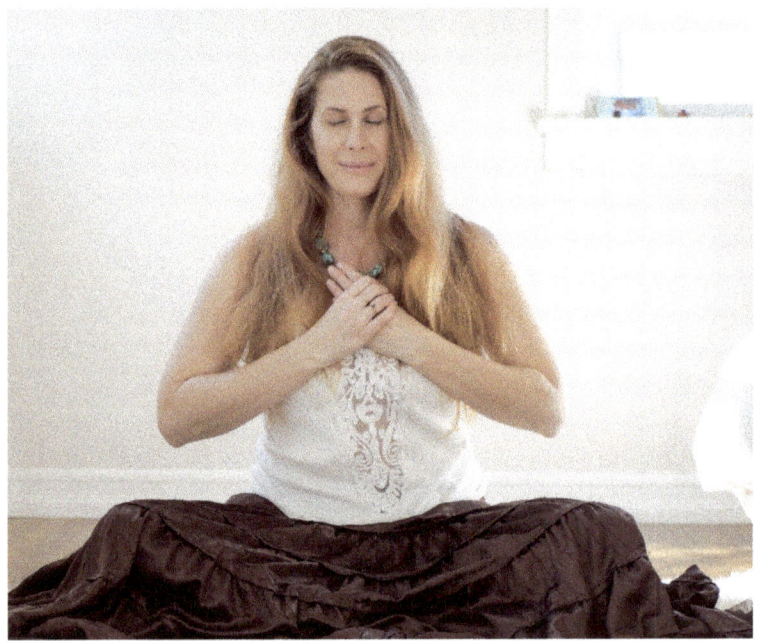

Sit comfortably in easy pose. Rest the back of the left hand in the palm of the right hand. The right thumb rests in the palm of the left hand and the left thumb crosses the right thumb.
The fingers of the right hand curve around the outside of the left hand.
Holding your hand in this way gives you peace and very secure feelings.

Place this mudra at your heart center with the palm side resting against your chest.

Meditate listening to "Dhan Dhan, Ram Das Gur" in your favorite version.

Begin with 11 minutes and gradually work up to 31 minutes.

To finish: inhale deeply and relax.

"The beauty in you is your spirit. The strength in you is your endurance. The intelligence in you is your vastness." Yogi Bhajan

Chapter 11
A Spiritual Teacher and Healer

"Knock, and He'll open the door. Vanish, And He'll make you shine like the sun. Fall, And He'll raise you to the heavens. Become nothing, And He'll turn you into everything."

    -Rumi

"Make yourself so happy so that when others look at you they become happy, too."

    -Yogi Bhajan

We have now arrived, metaphorically and literally, at the summit to Living in the Magic of Life. This is the last chapter of the book and therefore the highest point to climb to mentally. Spirituality for me is the way to swim through life's matrix in our individual journey at its highest level. Metaphorically speaking, to live in the Magic of Life is to see life from the highest peak in every moment. This chapter contains a beautiful vantage point to look around and to feel a sense of accomplishment in our own lives. As we take the time to integrate these memories, at this high point, we still our mind for a moment to appraise and to breathe for the sake of inner centeredness, inner space and with inner peace.

As I write this today, I must share what just took place. I was writing the last paragraph and someone knocked at my door. When I looked out, I saw a man with a child and a teenager holding a book. I immediately thought it was a Jehovah's Witness family and so I hesitated to open the door. Realizing that I was writing about Spirituality, it was probably important for me to open the door. Upon opening it, a man introduced himself and the two kids and explained how they use this time, around the holidays, to share the teachings to spread sustainable happiness.

He read Matthew, chapter 5, which talks about being welcome into the "kingdom" of happiness once you realize you are "poor" of Spirit. What a continuation of magical living this is for me. I could not have planned a better confirmation that living the in Magic of Life exists. To know that Living in the Magic of Life is synonymous with the Bible, feels like a nice gift for me because I have never read the Bible. I am glad to confirm to you that Spirituality is living in the Kingdom of

Heaven, which is living the in the Magic of Life and not being dogmatic about any one religion. It is the truth of Life and to this I say, thank you Magic for that interruption.

Inner openness to Spirituality requires a small commitment of beginning to use our eyes to perceive all our previous positions and situations as channels of growth towards our individual destinies. Rather than constantly looking back with regret at the things that hurt us, challenged us or forced us to grow, we commit to looking back at all of it with gratitude. Then it becomes alchemized and then we get to feel the Spirituality lift us up to higher circumstances. That commitment to your perception will constantly provide a supportive inner dialog like, "thank you for teaching me this or that lesson" as you re-program your subconscious mind. Let us become a cheerleader of sorts, where our mind gets programmed to motivate us in all moments.

This way of spiritually reacting or thinking is the strongest method for inner stamina and sustained happiness. All the metaphysical books and lectures, all the religious books, all the mystical texts and now science points us in the direction of Spirituality being not only the best way to live, but the way to "Heaven." Exactly as the example that Spirituality sent to my front door you will also receive messages dispersed throughout your life. It is beyond the ego's idea of Heaven because the ego will tell your mind to be competitive, separate from and stuck in the illusion.

A spiritual outlook on life comes from a deep inner experience of what all these texts and lectures talk about. Initiating the Spirituality from within will not only teach your subconscious mind, but it will raise the consciousness of the ego as well. Science calls it the quantum field, the Chinese call it Chi, the yogi's call it the chakra system and Kundalini energy, Kabbalah calls it Sefirot, but what all these explanations point to is simply an inner alignment with Source creation at all times. Most of us have no experience of feeling this because it was not taught to us in a non-religious way. I had to learn it through practicing Kundalini yoga to experience it and then on a mental level I understood, but we are arriving at the time when all of this is now available for us to feel.

Openness comes from having an open heart and no fear. Therefore, we must do the work individually that we each are called to do, whether it be chakra work, energy healing, alternative healing, yoga, Reiki, religion, mysticism or anything else that will put us into a place of living with an open heart. For some people getting to the daily work of healing and meditating to become open or to become Spiritual requires a big health scare, like cancer, getting older, losing a parent, or worse to wake us up to the reality that this life is meant to be fulfilling in a deep way. Once prompted by the challenge, we are forced to finally seek help because the pain of the big scare is too great for the mind and the body. The pain transforms us into being open to more possibility as if the pain was the medicine to break us open.

Spirituality is not religion. Spirituality is the underlying feeling we maintain while living life. Religion can get us to the feeling of Spirituality, but usually not from a preacher telling us what to do. No authority on the planet can force one into opening our perspective, but most of us do need a teacher. In the east a personal Teacher is well respected, while in the West a teacher is a government employee. A teacher can show us the work we need to do to heal, but the teacher will also tell you they cannot do the work for you. Humanity has so much healing to do from generations and lifetimes that we could each potentially be healing everyday for the rest of our lives.

The work simply feels difficult at first; like a new job can feel overwhelming the first day, but if you have an inspiring teacher, coach, or mentor to motivate you, they become a guiding light. If we could see past our aversion to doing work for inner healing and understand that the work is built into living the Spirituality of life, we would feel more accomplished with every passing day. Why pretend everything is fine, when deep down we all feel the need to ask for help. That is called an introvert or someone who is not vulnerable and not transparent. A teacher is like a mother cheering us on to continue our path with full acceptance of all our mistakes.

I have had many teachers and healers so far on my journey, which have become available right at the moment I felt darkest or overwhelmingly challenged. In the Western world, we do not understand that asking for help is empowering and not admitting we are weak. That is the misconception that I had for a long time. In fact, it was not until I became a Kundalini yoga teacher that I realized just how important having a teacher promises to be. Now that I see the improved impact on my life and my increased strength when asking for help, I understand the benefit of having a teacher; especially someone I admire or someone I believe can help me.

In the East it is apart of life to have a teacher or Guru. In the Kundalini yoga tradition, we were told that humanity no longer needs a Guru telling them what to do with every aspect of their lives. The secret has been revealed that humanity is meant to be our own Gurus. Although having a teacher teach you how to be your own Guru is the secret inherent in the yoga. Everyone gets to choose their own conclusions in their own time based on their experience of the work. Upon asking for guidance even in one area, we are benefitted. Teachers expect the very best of us and further our inner growth, our spiritual growth and our financial growth. Unless you have already done tons of work on your Self, asking for help is like receiving a Spiritual hint for your individual adventure.

This life is so special and it begs to be treated as a gift by blossoming for those of us who live fully in the Magic of Life. This requires so much consciousness and so much awareness to fully live in the moment. Otherwise, when living in the past or the future, the present moment cannot be appreciated and therefore, we miss the opportunity to create new by recreating more of the same. We will continue to live on the out of date old programming it will never feel better. Instead we must attune the subconscious program to upgrade with clarity. When we are mindful of the present moment, flowing in Spirituality, we become resourceful and choose, as a co-creator with Life, the future we wish to create.

My true desire is to share my story so that it creates a conversation between you and your memories from your life. Once you determine how far you have come, through self compassion, an underlying openness in your mind where the Light and the Magic can infuse your psyche will create your Heaven on Earth or Magical Life. How can I know with a profound confidence that sharing my story with you can create a change? I cannot be sure it will, but it is my service to help even one person turn on their inner Light and Spirituality.

I am sure that all my experiences were guiding me to be in this dimension of miracles, Magic and Spirituality creating my Heaven on Earth, but it would have been nice to read a book like this at fifteen. Based on my life experiences, I have learned to be confident in allowing my heart to make decisions because they are now informed by my intuition. I wish the same for friends, sisters, brothers, children, parents and humanity. This is what the ancient yogi's spoke of when illustrating the science of how humans are meant to live.

My contribution and my destiny are one, to share my life or at least start the conversation to open others up to speak about their lives. As I have heard before, "all paths lead us to the same destination" therefore, no matter how my life went, it is possible I would have arrived at this destination regardless. As you have read my life choices led me to my purpose and my destiny to become a Spiritual teacher and a healer; I am that I am. You may ask yourself, "Could she have made other choices to lead her somewhere else?" The answer would be, "yes, if you were me, you would have made other choices," but if you want to test me, do what I did and perhaps you will find your purpose, too? A purpose is not the goal to life. A purpose is something you do in your life where you feel like it is why you are on Earth every single time you do it. It is too beautiful to stand before my purpose in fear of taking the first step therefore, I stand before my purpose listening to my hearts' gifts and feeling the excitement of what is to come.

When we walk in the Magic of Life and we are living with our hearts open, our life choices become effortless and rewarding. It is our intuition leading us in the right direction in every moment. There is a special beauty and even if there are "painful moments," the finale promises expanded growth and evolution. After stepping into the entrance to our new paradigm, we will not go backwards, because this wormhole is becoming a tunnel of transformation that mimics a caterpillar entering metamorphosis to transform into a butterfly. Everything in my life has happened to lead me to this proverbial cocoon and the same is true for humanity. We are all at the end of our cocoon period as humans on this planet. All we need from here is to believe we have the strength and grit to be victorious.

With the unwavering belief in your path, the belief in your end result, the belief in your destiny and the decision to get there no matter what, the Magic will support you. Allow life to become like one long yoga class breathing deeply the entire time you feel through it. You have chosen your teacher to lead you. Naturally, the possibility exists of not loving every movement, every challenging pose or every awkward breath pattern, but remember that half the battle was simply getting to the class. You are alive now, so, the rest of the class is learning to listen to the suggestion or to modify. For it is prana that will carry the body and mind to keep up until the end when we are rewarded in savasana.

It is at the end of a yoga class, like when we sleep at the end of the day, where everything is integrated into our body temple. Integration is the reduction sauce of all your wisdom. We realize sooner or later that all the prodding, pain and poking of life was worth it. In fact after every yoga class, we feel we have even more patience, strength, grit and connection to Spirit than before we walked into class. A yoga class is the metaphor of life that you can carry with you into all parts of your life as you evolve, but a yoga class truly is a wonderful tool. Your destiny will feel so good because you will have listened to your inner voice the whole time.

If it sounds like I say this from experience, I am! I have only recently realized that life seems like one long yoga class with its deep lessons and intense awakenings slowly building one upon another after all these years. For example right after my abortion of the baby girl I wanted to name India, I used all my experience with yoga to navigate the pain and quickly breathe through it, but I didn't have a Spiritual teacher to tell me these types of deep pain take work to heal. I had people in my life that taught me how to think about it spiritually, but I was not ready to do it on my own. My biological father told me to name my daughter, Grace and to write her a note in gratitude. I looked at my dilemma in a Spiritual way, but at that point, I wasn't practicing Kundalini yoga and meditation. I was still too close to the pain and I was stuck in old painful thinking.

The fact that she was never born was like a thorn in my side providing me a dull pain in my heart, but after Kundalini yoga and meditation, I understood it was actually another gift of Spirituality. Magically it was not meant to stop my growth, as many of us can believe after such a painful life experience. It was a wake up call for advancement, but until the birth of my first-born son, Weston, I was not ready to dive into cleansing myself of the pain of aborting India. The first week Weston was alive, one night while holding him, I cried for the first time since my abortion, tears from all the stagnant emotion were released and I never felt more connected to Spirit. An inner healing and cleaning seemed to have finally occurred thanks to the relief of Weston being in my arms. I felt I could truly grieve that loss. I was reborn thanks to Weston. I believe he healed not only myself, but my husband, too. We both wanted to subconsciously heal from the deep loss of our first baby girl, India and with my new understanding of Spirituality (after becoming a student and certified to teach Kundalini yoga,) I see that India is now apart of the electro-magnetic field that surrounds my husband, my two boys and myself. That is a scientific definition of what it means to lead a Spiritual life.

I have always thought of babies as bringers of Spiritual abundance. Abundance of amazing experiences, of deep emotions, of prosperity, of ideas and a ton of Spiritual growth infused into the matrix. I believed this before having any kids as it felt logical, but now living through it, I understand it to an infinitely personal degree. Babies are said to be "a link between angels and man" author unknown. Or as Larry Barretto said, "babies are bits of stardust, blown from the hand of God." Our individual Spirit or soul always wants us to expand, enhance and grow stronger. It begins in pregnancy, but it is during birth that the "mother goes into the ethers to bring the soul of her child through the portal of the birth canal" Gurmukh Kaur Khalsa. Therefore, having babies is that decision from our soul to push us forward into a depth of Spiritual living that will make us evolve.

Children also push us forward in life from the sheer responsibility of caring for a being so full of Spirit, yet so helpless. They are so innocent and when taking care of a baby, this action brings out all the good, bad, ugly and everything else from within to transform us. The sleepless nights lend themselves to testing our character, our limits, and our Grace. Babies and children turn men and women into Mothers and Fathers. Somehow the phenomenon of having kids helps promote us to a deeper meaning in our life the way we never could before. Children guide us to where we are meant to go, do what we are meant to do and create what we are meant to create. I was led to Kundalini yoga based on my experiences from motherhood.

Praticing and teaching Hatha and Power yoga most of my young adult life helped me individually grow to an extent, but having a child consolidated my growth curve much faster. It forced me to look deeper into yogic philosophy to find Kundalini yoga and meditation, which zoomed me forward spiritually and mentally to a place of no return. When Weston was two I found myself disappointed with my power yoga practice and it was devastating because I was depressed. At that moment, I was about to receive one of the biggest surprises of my life. I had been praying and intending for something life enhancing to get me out of the darkness. My life was amazing and there was no reason for me to feel depressed because I was still enthralled in the energy of pure love becoming a mother. Something very big was missing. The energy of pure love led me to re-discover those teaching manuals from all those years before.

The Magic that this book is based on grasped me at the speed of light energy and I was pulled into exploring every word within these seemingly foreign teaching manuals. My curiosity grew with every word and page. When I began to follow the exercises, meditations and kriyas from the manuals, I began to feel different. This was another inner knowing that I had uncovered a real treasure. I was more than inspired because I was reborn.

Every Friday night I taught in the students in France and every Friday night I would feel so incredibly uplifted. That summer in 2015, I discovered living in the magic of life in a way that would change my destiny forever because I had uncovered my purpose. I worked up out of that depressed state to never return again. That is the power of this technology called Kundalini yoga and meditation. Whether I had slept or not because of my baby, it did not matter, I was happy for my life. I began to feel like I had the sun shinning from within. I developed an infinite energy inside of myself that was powering every relationship, every action, and every decision.

By mid-September, I found out that I was pregnant and this time it was a spontaneous pregnancy. Life had surprised me again with another Miracle thanks to Kundalini yoga. When my husband and I spoke earlier in August about having a second child, he expressed that he was not interested in having another baby using the medical route. I expressed that if that was our only way, we would decide a year from then. With the news of my second pregnancy, we were both surprised and shocked. It was not at all what we had planned, but underneath my plan, Spirit and the soul of Paxton had decided and I was excited.

From that summer until now, I recognized that living in the magic of life is the only way to live life for me. It is the energy of openness and it leaves room for miracles, surprises and total magic. I continued to live with this energy lifting me higher and higher as I went to L.A. to get prenatal Kundalini yoga from the best place, Golden Bridge Yoga. As I soaked myself in the magic of Gurmukh's presence and the beautiful prenatal Kundalini yoga available at Golden Bridge I understood my spirituality was giving me another chance to dream up a new birth experience. When Gurmukh told me to get her book, "Bountiful,

Blissful, Beautiful" and I did, she signed my copy and told me how blessed I was and that my baby would be as well.

Still riding high on the energy of her presence, I went back to France with an inner fervor to teach, to share and to create a deeper spiritual space inside of me for my baby. I added prenatal Kundalini yoga for pregnant women to inspire them to have conscious birth experiences. Plus, it was comforting and inspiring for the pregnant women to have a yoga teacher who was also pregnant alongside of them. I decided to have a natural birth at home in a birthing pool and my determination mixed with the inner energy of magic, gave me the empowerment I needed to succeed. In May of 2016, I gave birth to Paxton at home in a birthing pool and it was filmed as part of a documentary about natural births in France; which are illegal.

Therefore, a year after discovering Kundalini yoga and meditation I was yet again living through miracles right before my eyes. I am so grateful to Kundalini yoga and the magic of life for gifting me with such abundance and purpose in my lifetime. Having the experience of giving birth at home to a healthy, happy and incredible kundalini baby boy, gave me a full spectrum glimpse into my destiny. When Paxton was six months old and I began the last Teachers Training Golden Bridge Santa Monica would provide I knew I was living my destiny.

Literally every single thing I learned in teachers training was information I was seeking my whole childhood. It is almost as if I had known all my life that I was meant to acquire the vast quantity of information downloaded during teachers training. Perhaps even, that I had "been a Kundalini yoga practitioner in a past life", as Gurmukh and Gurushabd recounted during the training. I am awake now to the fact that I was given two opportunities to begin Kundalini yoga early on in my life, but I was not ready then. This technology is strong for healing all the layers of deep pain within like an onion when we truly commit to ourselves.

I was not ready at seventeen when my boyfriend's mother took me. I was not ready at twenty-one when my acting school friend Julie Greyfus introduced me to Gurmukh. Apparently, I needed more life experience such as an auto-immune dis-order, losing a baby, having a baby, depression and all the other self-healing I was doing for so many years to prepare me for the profound healing that the technology of Kundalini yoga provides. Becoming certified in Kundalini yoga has chisled me into a Spiritual teacher, a golden light leader and a golden light goddess healer. I have always had Spirituality inside of me asking to come out, but without being able to let it lead my life until now.

Teaching five times a week along with my own practice, I have awakened to my subtle abilities in the realm of healing. I had to look up what it meant to be a clairsentient. I am so grateful and relieved to finally uncover the reason I have felt energy my whole life. I have discovered my gifts and I am excited to begin to help others realize their inner gifts. Our gifts no longer need go shuffled under the rug, discounted, or be killed or accused of being a "witch" with gifts like these. These gifts are natural for all humanity to uncover within and to be enhanced.

For it is with these abilities that we should be honored and teach compassion for humankind. The new paradigm of learning our gifts and sharing them is for all our futures. How do I know this? I know this because I feel it within myself. It is our future because it has already been in the past. And I know this because we are in the Age of Aquarius where all truth is coming to the surface and all negativity, fear, darkness and false ways of living are exploding out of the surface like a pimple begging to be healed. Once our humanity can heal its' own fears, greed and negativity then every human will know the truth. The Butterfly Effect of this type of awakening will manifest a total healing of beautiful Mother Earth so quick that our planet can return to its original Garden of Eden.

Our perspectives will self correct so that we can see the truth of what we are doing here. The beauty of darkness and the depth of one's darkness is just an example of how deeply one can feel the light. It is similar to the energy of Yin and Yang from Chinese medicine, which is another way of describing the polarity of this dimension. The darkness is the other side of the coin of light. If we did not know sadness, we would not know happiness. And our future is to know the truth, which is that happiness is possible and moreover a scientific fact for all beings.

The Dalai Lama says, "the more compassionate our mind is, the better our brain functions…compassion gives us inner strength." What is compassion, but an awakening of our inner self-love projected out onto others. This is my method of describing it and I am starting to believe that despite all the confusion about the emotion of love, if we can get truly conscious, then we can discover that love is simply energy. It is starting to become very clear for me that God=Love. Instead of praying to God, let's pray to Love. Let us imagine that when people in Spiritual positions say, "we are all Gods and Goddesses," they are really saying we are Love." It can be better understood as an inner Love we feel inside our mind and body. I found another quote from the bible from John 4:16. "God is Love; and he who abides in Love abides in God and God abides in him."

Spirituality is truly a location that the mind must experience and live within. Once we can feel it and truly experience it, than we can continually become the empty vacuum ready to be filled up. We are to constantly empty ourselves of all our stuff, appointments, school start times, obligations, work, play, fun, etc. and give it to the Magic. Once we live in the Magic of Life Spirit will take care of it all. It is a co-creation of sorts and once we are empty of the worry, Spirit can make it all clear. Living in the Magic of Life wants you to jump into its energy and prove itself to you, but you have to ask.

Look at it like a prayer that you release into the atmosphere. We are taught to pray to God, but what if we began to replace God with Magic. Do you remember being in love with someone or something? When we are "in love," we are in our natural divine state and our hearts are open to all the Magic that life has to offer. We get married because of the Magic we feel deep inside. We must realize that we are worth that kind of love and work, learn, and heal until we discover how to always live in the Magic.

It also confirms for me that we must remember that we are one. I spoke earlier about how we are all connected and how everything in the matrix of life is connected. So, if you are someone who believes in God, than you have certainly heard that God includes everything. Therefore if we are all connected and everything is God, than we are all a piece of this God-like divinity that is energy. When we feel this divine energy, we feel a super humanness and we begin to notice the flowers and we feel that life is magical. If we can feel that way some of the time, than we can feel that way all of the time. We can continue to smell the flowers and remain open to the magic of life even through tragedy, pain, or challenging moments. We go through those moments of fear, pain and darkness to crawl out the other side as stronger people, just like in the movies, even more open and glued to the feeling of magic.

As you have seen by now, I have provided some meditations in the book for you to do your own explorations into Spiritual work for yourself. This last meditation is no different and no less amazing towards transforming your life into a Magical life. We must be courageous to do the inner work in order to harvest the amazing rewards. As I have attempted to explain, you are the artist of your own life so, go out there and paint it colorfully with a ton of sparkly magic.

Meditation:
Hast Kriya "Earth To Heavens"

Sit in easy pose with your eyes closed. Extend your Jupiter finger on both hands.

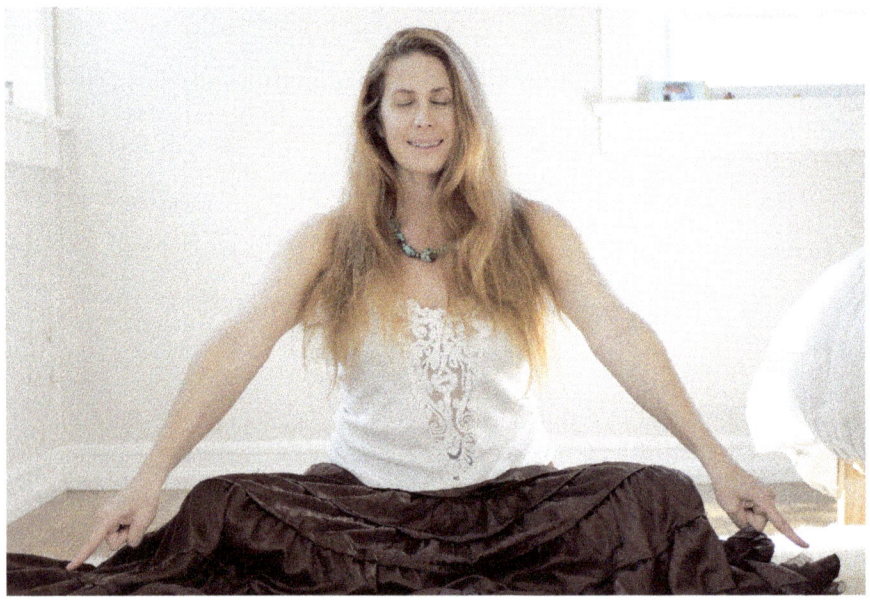

Lock the fingers down with your thumbs.
Time your movements to the song, "sat nam wahe guru."
Touch your Jupiter fingers to the floor on either side of you on "Sat."
Then on "Nam" touch the Jupiter fingers together over the top of your head 6-12 inches.

Keep going in this way for up to 22 minutes.
Start with 11 minutes.

This kriya renews the nervous system and can heal nerve pain and sciatica.

It is so powerful it can hold the Hand of God; so powerful, it can hold the hand of death.

"Sat Nam Wahe Guru" is a Jupiter mantra. The most graceful power and knowledge comes from Jupiter. Jupiter controls the medulla oblongata, the neurological center of the brain, and the three rings of the brain stem.

If you do this Kriya for 22 minutes a day, you will change your personality. Power will descend from above and clean you out.

"We are all together in the One Creator's Consciousness."
-Yogi Bhajan

www.ingramcontent.com/pod-product-compliance
Lightning Source LLC
Chambersburg PA
CBHW062026290426

44108CB00025B/2797